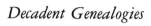

Decadent Genealogies

Decadent Genealogies

THE RHETORIC OF SICKNESS FROM
BAUDELAIRE TO D'ANNUNZIO

BARBARA SPACKMAN

Cornell University Press

ITHACA AND LONDON

First published 1989 by Cornell University Press.

International Standard Book Number 0-8014-2290-6
Library of Congress Catalog Card Number 89-7303
Printed in the United States of America
Librarians: Library of Congress cataloging information
appears on the last page of the book.

The paper in this book is acid-free and meets the guidelines for permanence and durability of the Committee on Production Guidelines for Book Longevity of the Council on Library Resources.

Contents

Preface

The nineteenth-century theorization of mental illness passed first through the sick body of the degenerate: sick bodies produced sick thought. As a scientific model, pre-Freudian theories of degeneration enjoyed a brief, though influential, reign. As a set of rhetorical strategies with which to describe not only sick bodies and their thoughts but also social classes, political positions, genders, and even literary texts, those theories continued to hold sway well into the twentieth century. Thus, though the texts that bear the names of Cesare Lombroso, Friedrich Nietzsche, Benedetto Croce, Max Nordau, Antonio Gramsci, G. A. Borgese, Georg Lukács, Charles Baudelaire, J. K. Huysmans, Sigmund Freud, and Gabriele D'Annunzio clearly occupy different ideological camps and even different centuries, they are nonetheless familial in their adoption of what might be called the *rhétorique obsédante* of the nineteenth century: the rhetoric of sickness and health, decay and degeneration, pathology and normalcy. This book attempts to chart the changing ideological inflections of that rhetoric as the hands that wield it change, as it moves from discipline to discipline, from genre to genre. A selection of D'Annunzio's prose works constitutes the point of departure and the final destination of a genealogical itinerary that takes into consideration the scientific intertext to literary and critical texts, as well as the French subtext to Italian "decadence."

Decadent writers place themselves on the side of pathology and valorize physiological ills and alteration as the origin of psychic alterity. The decadent rhetoric of sickness embraces and exalts the counternatural as an opening onto the unconscious, an alibi for alterity. Literary critics, instead, first launch their antidecadent attack from an island of normalcy, an island located in the pre-Freudian criminological intertext to the language of criticism. The first chapter examines the roots of antidecadent and anti-D'Annunzian criticism in the medicolegal studies of Cesare Lombroso and their first "literary" application in Max Nordau. D'Annunzio's texts have been lacerated by two schools that are presumably at ideological odds with each other: Crocean idealism and the current of Marxist criticism which favors "realistic" narrative. These schools concur in surprising ways. For Lukács, decadent writers represent an "overturning of values"; for Croce, theirs is "the great industry of emptiness," and Giovanni Pascoli, Antonio Fogazzaro, and D'Annunzio are three "neurotics." Lukács sees a "vital struggle between health and decay" in art and finds decadent art battling on the wrong side. Gramsci declares that "D'Annunzio was the Italian people's last bout of sickness." Reading the literary text as a symptom of a diseased body, these critics condemn the text as morally and politically reprehensible, but their condemnation cannot hastily be attributed to a shared political stance, and even less to shared aesthetic theories. The chapter links these condemnations to the politics and rhetoric of Cesare Lombroso's criminological studies and Max Nordau's *Degeneration*. When these texts are read together, a different perspective appears. The critics' antipathy to D'Annunzio fixes upon erotic discourse (rather than, say, political discourse or even D'Annunzio's problematic relationship to fascism) as a locus of pathology; what these critics object to is a lack of "virility." This preoccupation appears in Lombroso's texts as well, where degeneration is, finally, de*gender*ation. And it can be said to stand at the very roots of decadentism itself, for when Anatole Baju founded the journal *Le Décadent*, its call to arms was "Man becomes more refined, more feminine, more divine." The attacks on the decadents thus represent less an analysis of the literary text than an imposition of an opposing ideology *onto* the text.

Eviration and feminization are in fact constitutive elements of the decadent rhetoric of sickness. In Chapter 2 I examine Baudelaire's essay *Le peintre de la vie moderne*, novels of J. K. Huysmans

and D'Annunzio—*A rebours* and *Il piacere*—and Nietzsche's preface
to the second edition of *The Gay Science*. Convalescence as the scene
of artistic and philosophic creation is an ideologeme of decadent
texts, a narrative that lies between texts. The painter Constantin
Guys in *Le peintre de la vie moderne* stands as legitimating father of
the aesthete Des Esseintes in *A rebours*, the failed poet Andrea
Sperelli in *Il piacere*, and the narrator of the 1886 preface to *The
Gay Science*. All are convalescent and participate in what I call a
Baudelairean rhetoric of sickness. This Baudelairean convalescent
is the site of an intersection between psychology and physiology;
lingering sickness, fevers, and congestion are the ground of a
new consciousness, a new interpretation of the body's relation to
thought. In all four of these texts, that attempt at a new interpretation comes into being through a feminization of the male "protagonist," who thus discovers a ventriloquistic mode of speech in which
the body spoken through is necessarily a "woman's" body.

To arrive at this ventriloquist movement, the convalescent narrative follows certain steps. The convalescent is socially and topo-
graphically dislocated and occupies a liminal position even when,
as in the case of Constantin Guys, he is described as "the man of
the crowd." Eviration and a death of desire occur upon passage into
the state of convalescence. This eviration is clearly marked in Des
Esseintes's case—a dinner mourning the death of his virility is
given on the eve of his withdrawal into solitude—and is alluded
to in descriptions of the convalescent as child in Baudelaire and
D'Annunzio. Woman is expelled from the scene of convalescence.
This expulsion is not, however, the expulsion of her attributes.
Indeed, woman is expelled in order to abstract her qualities and
reassign them to the evirated convalescent himself. Convalescence
is figured as a sort of secular conversion: the old woman is expelled
in order that the new woman may be put on, that the converted
convalescent may assume a feminine guise. The resultant physiological ambiguity of the convalescent opens the way to figures of
androgyny and hermaphroditism: in Baudelaire's case, to a discussion of the androgyny of genius; in D'Annunzio's and Nietzsche's,
to the description of poetic and philosophic production as giving
birth. This occupation of the woman's body is both the decadent's
profession and the means by which he appropriates alterity.

Chapter 3 analyzes scenes of convalescence in D'Annunzio's *Terra vergine, Le novelle della Pescara,* and *L'Innocente,* but these are "Lombrosian" convalescences, which are the scene not of conversion to artistic creation and ventriloquism, but rather of hysterical conversion. Not coincidentally, the diseased character is female and of the lower class, in contrast to the upper-class male convalescent of Chapter 2. While the Baudelairean rhetoric converts symptoms into signs that the subject himself is able to read, the Lombrosian rhetoric reduces psychic activity to the tyranny of the symptom. Chapter 3 creates a dialogue between *Le novelle delle Pescara* and the *Studies on Hysteria* of Sigmund Freud and Josef Breuer by analyzing the narrative structure of Freud's clinical studies in relation to that of D'Annunzio's fiction. In the early Freud, hypnosis serves to induce the traits of convalescence by inducing forgetfulness; it is here that Freud begins to read and translate what he calls the "pictographic script" of the hysteric's body. The tales of "La vergine Orsola" and "La vergine Anna" follow a similar itinerary. The woman's body is spoken through once again, but it is not she who speaks; she is not a ventriloquist but a hysteric who assumes postures recorded by Freud's predecessor Jean-Martin Charcot.

A different approach is reserved for the male Lombrosian convalescent. In *L'Innocente,* another aspect of Baudelaire's influence is filtered through the Lombrosian rhetoric, for both the texts that bear his signature and Baudelaire *himself* as text enter the semiosis of decadence. When his fatal illness is mythified (by Lombroso as well as by writers such as Maurice Barrès) as the most horrifying of all writer's fates, Baudelaire becomes a sign. This aspect of Baudelairean "influenza" is filtered through the Lombrosian rhetoric, and ideological sympathy threatens to become physiological similarity. In fact, Lombroso's followers recognized *L'Innocente* as a faithful representation of a criminal *alienato.* But though the narrator's self-diagnosis is drawn from Lombroso, his discourse is structured by mechanisms that Freud will claim are proper to oneiric discourse and the work of censorship: negation, condensation, and displacement. When so read, *L'Innocente* turns out to constitute, both thematically and rhetorically, a prereading of the Freudian account of Oedipus. What Freud will see as the son's desire to kill the father appears here as the father's desire to kill the son projected onto the son, for the narrator commits parricide and infanticide in one condensed stroke.

Chapter 4 analyzes the rhetoric of sickness as applied to the upper-class female body. Neither Baudelairean nor Lombrosian, it might be labeled specifically D'Annunzian, for it constitutes the erotic discourse of the *Romanzi della Rosa* trilogy and the basis for erotic discourse in D'Annunzio's later works. Here disease seems to constitute a prohibition that must be transgressed in order that the discourse be erotic. It is, in fact, a commonplace of D'Annunzian criticism that these diseases represent a prohibition, but naturalistic explanations are inadequate, for none of these diseases is, medically speaking, communicable. Convalescents appear once again, though the maladies from which they "recover" are figured as sacred and demonic: epilepsy, gynecological ills, "the hysterical demon." Another critical commonplace is the notion that sickness renders the woman a ready-made victim of the male protagonist's sadistic desires; such an interpretation is, in fact, clearly stated in the texts themselves. I argue, instead, that these "female troubles" represent a different sort of contagion: the contagion of castration. The novels of the trilogy narrativize the logic of fetishism: repeated scenes in which the nature of woman's physiology is "unveiled" are followed by disbelief and disavowal. The topos of the enchantress-turned-hag so prevalent in *Il piacere* is but the thematic introduction to the textual fetishism of *L'Innocente*, where *fallo* (in Italian, at once the emblem of the virile member or the organ itself; an error or equivocation; a defect, failing, or imperfection; a sin or offense) suspends the decision between present and absent phallus and stands for the fetishist's simultaneous denial and affirmation of castration, at the same time as it names itself as equivocation. In *La Gioconda*, a narrative of mutilation once again sets in motion the logic of fetishism. This Medusan moment is the consequence of the decadents' occupation of the woman's body, and necessarily haunts these texts in which eviration represents a desired state.

Unless otherwise noted, all translations in this book are mine. The choice of what to include in the original and what to include only in translation was a difficult one. In the best of all possible worlds, all texts would be cited in the original and followed by a translation. This not being the case, I have adopted the following criteria: (1) French and Italian texts dealt with as primary sources (a category that includes the writings of Cesare Lombroso and those

of the D'Annunzian critics cited in Chapter 1) are given both in
the original and in translation; (2) French and Italian texts cited as
secondary sources are given only in translation; (3) since the German
texts I cite all exist in standard translations, they are given in
translation with key words and phrases interpolated when necessary. In developing my translations of D'Annunzio's work, I consulted the following: *Tales of My Native Town*, trans. Rafael Mantel-
lini (New York: Doubleday, 1920); *The Child of Pleasure*, trans.
Georgina Harding, verses translated by Arthur Symons (Boston:
L. C. Page, 1898); *The Intruder*, trans. Arthur Hornblow (New
York: George G. Richmond, 1898); *The Triumph of Death*, trans.
Arthur Hornblow (New York: Boni and Liveright, 1923); *Gioconda*, trans. Arthur Symons (New York: R. H. Russell, 1902).

The writing of this book was greatly aided in its early stages by
a grant from the Mrs. Giles Whiting Foundation and given a final
boost by a quarter's leave from Northwestern University.

A portion of Chapter 2 appeared as "Nietzsche, D'Annunzio,
and the Scene of Convalescence" in *Stanford Italian Review* 6.1–2
(1986): 141–57, and a condensed version of the section "Prometheus and Pandora" appeared as "Pandora's Box" in *Quaderni Dannunziani* 3–4 (1988): 61–73. Professor Pietro Gibellini and the
Fondazione del Vittoriale degli Italiani have kindly granted me
permission to quote and translate from *Tutte le opere di Gabriele
D'Annunzio*.

The idea for this book had its origins in a seminar on decadentism
taught by Paolo Valesio. In spite of ideological disagreement, he
has been unfailingly generous with his considerable learning, critical insights, and encouragement. I also thank John Freccero for his
sensitive reading at an early stage and for his support on numerous
occasions.

A number of friends and colleagues have read and reread this
book. Alice Y. Kaplan's comments on an early version were extremely helpful. I am grateful to Antonella Ansani, Margaret
Morton, Ann Mullaney, and Juliana Schiesari, who, at different
moments, have read portions of the manuscript and urged me on.
Albert R. Ascoli has been not only an astute critic of the later
stages of the manuscript but also a generous colleague and friend.
Jeffrey Schnapp's attentive reading of the manuscript as it neared

its final form gave me the inspiration I needed to complete it. I owe very warm thanks to Carla Freccero, Nancy Harrowitz, and especially Marilyn Migiel; they have suffered through every version of this book, and their criticisms, suggestions, and questions have been as invaluable as their friendship. Their presence (epistolary, telephonic, electronic, and sometimes even in the flesh) has made this a better book than it might otherwise have been. I am more than grateful to my parents for having believed in me, no matter what. Finally, I thank Andrzej Warminski: for readings past and future.

BARBARA SPACKMAN

Chicago

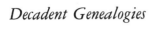

Decadent Genealogies

[1] *The Island of Normalcy*

As a critical gesture, the diagnosis of "sickness" reduces the work of the intellect to the twitches of a body jolted by nerve spasms, poisoned by disease. The literary text, rather than a work of sign production, becomes a set of symptoms not (*not*, rather than *un*-) consciously produced. In its concern for cure, such a critical discourse traces the symptoms back to the subjects who display them and finds those subjects off-center, contaminated by physiology, irrational, and even criminal. Yet the question asked is not *who* produced a text but *what*—what disease, what atavistic deformity, what hereditary fault. Something speaks through the subject, but in the pre-Freudian texts that are the most ambitious proponents of this discourse, it is not language, not yet the unconscious. Behind the disturbed syntax, the disturbing contents of decadent texts, there hides a diseased, degenerate body. Post-Freudian symptomatic readings rely on an analysis of psychic mechanisms to interpret texts; nineteenth-century medicolegal anthropological studies (as their authors call them) ground their interpretive code on a description of somatic reactions, not the unconscious. These pre-Freudian texts are as blissfully unaware of that dark continent as they are of disciplinary boundaries. When the ideologeme of sickness recurs in the post-Freudian literary-critical condemnation of decadentism, a persistent "ignorance" of the unconscious becomes instead a repudiation of it.

Pre-Freudian, post-Freudian—perhaps the very distinction should be put into question. Freud himself begins to eavesdrop on the unconscious when hysteria speaks: "It was on this place that her father used to rest his leg every morning, while she renewed the bandage round it, for it was badly swollen. This must have happened a good hundred times, yet she had not noticed the connection till now. In this way she gave me the explanation that I needed of the emergence of what was an atypical hysterogenic zone. Further, her painful legs began to 'join in the conversation' (mitsprechen) during our analyses."[1] Fräulein Elizabeth von R., whose talking legs launched a career, could not be hypnotized, but Freud, by resting his hand upon her head, could hear the body talk. Psychoanalysis rests on the somatic compliance unique to hysteria, is founded on the hysterical woman's symptom. Freud was not alone in listening to the body talk (Max Nordau thought he heard it loud and clear) or in privileging the woman's symptom as a matrix for his theory (Cesare Lombroso measured both skull and hymen). But whereas for psychoanalytic discourse it is the psychic event that requests compliance of the body, for the "average" psychiatric text of the late nineteenth century it is physiological disease and alteration that cause psychic events. A reversal of the causal chain, a turning of the topos of cause and effect, allowed Freud to endure, to create his field, while the opposing view continued to hold sway, not in psychiatry or medicine but in the literary criticism that castigates decadent writers.[2]

A genealogy of that literary criticism must, if only as a beginning, rescue at least one such "loser" from the dust clouds of mediocrity. Of course, neither Cesare Lombroso (who considered himself a criminological psychiatrist) nor his follower Max Nordau (both physician and critic) has gone unacknowledged as a critic of decadence, but recognition has assumed the form of dismissive exclamations, hyperboles devoted to their "stupidity."[3] The very

1. Sigmund Freud and Josef Breuer, *Studies on Hysteria*, vol. 2 of *The Standard Edition of the Complete Psychological Works of Sigmund Freud*, trans. James Strachey (London: Hogarth Press and the Institute of Psychoanalysis, 1956), 148.

2. For a discussion of Freud's relation to the alienists' concept of degeneration in the context of the history of ideas, see Sander Gilman, *Difference and Pathology* (Ithaca: Cornell University Press, 1985), esp. 191–216, "Sexology, Psychoanalysis, and Degeneration."

3. Typical is the description of nineteenth-century medical texts, including

evaluation of "stupidity," however, is a coordinate of the ideolo-geme it claims to supersede. Sickness, as I have said, destroys the intellect; the same critics who dismiss Lombroso and Nordau as "stupid" are quick to tell us that D'Annunzio had no "ideas." By refusing to take average sign production (and, in this case, the critics' own genealogy) seriously, such criticism retains this "stu-pidity" and transforms it into a symptom (now post-Freudian) of which it is unaware. Anti-D'Annunzian criticism, almost a genre in itself, obsessively repeats the same practices that excite its scorn for Nordau: it denies and deeply mistrusts the figurality of lan-guage; it willfully ignores the distinction between author and protagonist, author and text; it castrates the literary text in order to accuse it of impotence.

Such a refusal to read the "average" signs that surround and contextualize the signs privileged by the literary tradition may be countered by another sort of refusal. The critic, writes Paolo Valesio, "should refuse ideological hierarchies, and he should look at every literary text as part of a contexture of 'average' texts whose study is necessary in order to understand the text at issue as a socially conditioned object of sign production."[4] An average text, from this point of view, is one that marks no epistemological break as recognized by cultural criticism, one that has not been institutionalized as required reading in the history of a national literature or culture. An average text is one that has lost the round of literary fisticuffs from which the "great writers" of its age emerge.

allusions to Lombroso and Nordau, in A. E. Carter, *The Idea of Decadence in French Literature, 1830–1900* (Toronto: University of Toronto Press, 1958). In his chapter "Nerve Storms and Bad Heredity," Carter discusses French texts diagnostic of *dégénérescence*, which Lombroso knew and quoted extensively: "It must be admitted that these treatises make heavy reading nowadays. They occupy a worthy place in the history of psychiatry, but their absurdity as literary criticism is self-evident, and did not escape contemporary censure. None of the doctors, whatever their eminence in pathology, had much flair in the field of aesthetics. Irony, *blague,* and all the delicate shades of meaning and intention slipped through their heavy fingers like minnows. Nordau was particularly obtuse, and Moreau's incomprehension almost passes belief" (68). See also Robert Mitchell, "The Deliquescence of Decadence: Floupette's Eclectic Target," *Nineteenth-Century French Studies* 9 (Spring–Summer 1981): 247–56.

   4. Paolo Valesio, "The Practice of Literary Semiotics: A Theoretical Pro-posal," *Point of Contact/Punto de Contacto* 5 (April–May 1978): 19.

In approaching the average text, we find before us ideological screens that have rendered it "ridiculous," "unreadable," labeled it (and now I speak of D'Annunzio rather than Lombroso) kitsch. In fact, both Lombroso and D'Annunzio have been "averaged" if we understand "averaging" as the imposition of such extraordinarily opaque screens. In a sense, I "average" them once again, for the real subject of this book is less the novelistic production of Gabriele D'Annunzio than the changing ideological inflections of the decadent rhetoric of sickness. But here a leveling of texts, a refusal to remain within an individual text, is ventured in the hope of delineating the possibilities and limitations of a particular discursive formation, of reading the unreadable.

Uncovering the "average" intertext to literary criticism is, to some extent, a Foucauldian task; indeed, Foucault himself is no stranger to this land. With his surveyor's eye he has, in *The Birth of the Clinic,* mapped the territory discovered by the discipline of pathological anatomy. In the late eighteenth century, according to Foucault, disease was newly defined as a deviation internal to life, rather than a punitive will that attacks life from without.[5] The interdependence of the opposition between "sickness" and "health," between "pathological" and "normal," is thus made visible:

> Furthermore, the prestige of the sciences of life in the nineteenth century, their role as a model, especially in the human sciences, is linked originally not with the comprehensive, transferable character of biological concepts, but, rather, with the fact that these concepts were arranged in a space whose profound structure responded to the healthy/morbid opposition. When one spoke of the life of groups and societies, of the life of the race, or even of the 'psychological life,' one did not think first of the internal structure of the *organized being* but of the *medical bipolarity of the normal and the pathological.*

5. The latter conception, though no longer accepted as scientific, remains available as literature, as a metaphor of social disintegration or divine wrath. From Boccaccio to Manzoni to Camus, it loses none of its potency. It is predominantly this aspect that Susan Sontag examines in *Illness as Metaphor* (New York: Farrar, Straus and Giroux, 1977) and Gian Paolo Biasin highlights in *Literary Diseases: Theme and Metaphor in the Italian Novel* (Austin: University of Texas Press, 1975).

Consciousness lives because it can be altered, maimed, di-
verted from its course, paralysed; societies live because there
are sick declining societies, and healthy expanding ones.[6]

A "new" opposition magnetically reorders the linguistic expression
of scientific, literary, and political observations; a contagious rhetoric spreads from the body to the already-made topos of the body
politic. The very epithet "decadent," uttered first by critics en-
camped on an island of normalcy, is filtered through a positivistic
progressive ideology that can define itself only against a negative
regressive pole. When writers accept the epithet, when Anatole
Baju titles his literary magazine *Le Décadent*, it is to make a
statement both semiotic and ideological.[7] "Le Décadent" collapses
the opposition to an identity, denies the existence of an isle of
health and of the clear-eyed ones who claim to reside there. There
is only decadence, only sickness, and only those who welcome it
can represent "progress": "Déjà les décadents, précurseurs de la
société future, se rapprochent beaucoup du type idéal de la
perfection. . . . L'homme s'affine, se féminise, se divinise" ["Precursors of future society, the decadents are already quite close to
the ideal type of perfection. . . . Man becomes more refined, more
feminine, more divine"].[8] Science speaks a language of decay and
degeneration, progressive and regressive evolution. Literature and
criticism, too, speak such a language, but whereas Foucault emphasizes the regularities of this formation, creating a finely etched
monolith bordered by clifflike discontinuities, I hope to read the
etchings within the monolith, to trace the battles fought within
the space created by the rhetoric of sickness. Literature and science
and criticism all speak through this rhetoric, yes, but they do not
say the same thing.

6. Michel Foucault, *The Birth of the Clinic,* trans. A. M. Sheridan Smith
(New York: Vintage Books, 1975), 35; trans. of *La naissance de la clinique* (Paris:
Presses Universitaires de France, 1963).

7. For a history of the term *décadent,* see Louis Marquèze-Pouey, *Le mouve-
ment décadent en France* (Paris: Presses Universitaires de France, 1986), and
Richard Gilman, *Decadence: The Strange Life of an Epithet* (New York: Farrar,
Straus and Giroux, 1975).

8. Pierre Vareilles, "Le progrès," in *Le Décadent,* ed. Anatole Baju, no. 1
(10 April 1886); facsimile edition (Paris: L'Arche du Livre, 1970–73), n.p.

As the example of *Le Décadent* suggests, a rhetoric of sickness does not automatically presuppose a rhetoric of health. Ideological inflections begin to be visible when we map the boundaries of discourse, the closures imposed upon the admissible and the imaginable.[9] Health as a "logical" opposite of sickness appears in the criticism condemning decadence, where it stands for alternative practice, be it the realist novel (Lukács), the classicism of Giosuè Carducci (Croce), or the novels of Harriet Beecher Stowe (Nordau). Lukács is most straightforward in the essay "Healthy or Sick Art?": "Literary and art history is a mass graveyard where many artists of talent rest in deserved oblivion because they neither sought nor found any association to the problems of advancing humanity and did not set themselves on the right side in the vital struggle between health and decay." Decadents are decadent not because they depict illness and decay but because they do not recognize the existence of health, of the social sphere that would reunite the alienated writer to the progressive forces of history. Sickness, then, is a reactionary mode of insertion into the class struggle; sickness, writes Lukács, "produces a complete overturning of values." Though "sick art" may have its dialectical moment in the sun (Lukács cites only *Antigone* as an example), it is destined for the dust heap of history, while "healthy art" is a "reflection of the lasting truth of human relationships."[10] Max Nordau would seem to be a kindred spirit; the doctor offers his own prescription in "Prognosis," the penultimate chapter of *Degeneration:*

> We stand now in the midst of a severe mental epidemic; of a sort of black death of degeneration and hysteria, and it is natural that we should ask anxiously on all sides: "What is to come next?" . . . Art cannot take any side in politics, nor is it its business to find and propose solutions to economic questions. Its task is to represent the eternally human causes

9. For a fuller discussion of ideological closure, see Fredric Jameson, *The Political Unconscious* (Ithaca: Cornell University Press, 1981), esp. the opening chapter. See also Pierre Macherey, *A Theory of Literary Production,* trans. Geoffrey Wall (Boston: Routledge and Kegan Paul, 1978); trans. of *Pour une théorie de la production littéraire* (Paris: Maspero, 1974).

10. Georg Lukács, "Healthy or Sick Art?" in *Writer and Critic,* ed. and trans. Arthur D. Kahn (New York: Grosset and Dunlap, 1971), 109, 107, 104.

of the socialist movement, the suffering of the poor, their yearning after happiness, their struggle against hostile forces in Nature and in the social mechanism, and their mighty elevation from the abyss into a higher mental and moral atmosphere.[11]

Nordau, the physician, ideologizes the terms of his trade, his (pre-Freudian) physiology of hysteria, to diagnose the decadents vituperatively; Lukács, the metaphysician, attempts to "elevate" those terms to metaphysical categories. That attempt only emphasizes their most polemical and still recent history, their centrality in nineteenth-century forensic medicine, their ideologization in the literary battle over decadence, degeneration, and progress. Lukács's historical perspective gropes for expression in a language that, on one hand, recalls recent history and, on the other, presents itself as an ahistorical equivalent of "good" and "evil." His essay becomes an arena of violent clash between a rhetoric of class struggle and a rhetoric of sickness.

But why speak of clash? Nordau too prescribes the social mission of art as the road to health. Were not this rhetoric of sickness and that of class struggle perhaps spawned together, not warring brothers but brothers fighting the same battle? No, quite the contrary. Both Marxism and the social science of criminology can be seen as responses to the appearance of an urban proletariat; both deplore the present, but their analyses of causes and proposals for solutions are at odds. The discourse of what Lombroso calls legal psychiatry excludes revolution from the admissible and the imaginable; it is an ideology of evolutionary, not revolutionary, change. Degenerates, graphomaniacs, hysterics, epileptics, and the insane are examples of regressive evolution, the end of a line destined to die out. Socialism, yes, but no "anarchists,"[12] please; reform, but

11. Max Nordau, *Degeneration*, 6th ed. (New York: D. Appleton, 1895), 537, 546; trans. of *Entartung*, 2d ed. (Berlin: C. Duncker, 1892–93), hereafter cited in the text. The text bears a dedication to "Caesar Lombroso, Professor of Psychiatry and Forensic Medicine at the Royal University of Turin. By the Author."

12. While Lombroso does refer to historical figures, citing Peter Kropotkin and Mikhail Bakunin, as well as many less well known political assassins and criminals, as examples of anarchist physiology and psychology, his broad notion

no bloody uprisings: "But all these talks about sunrise, the dawn, the new land, etc., are only the twaddle of degenerates incapable of thought. The idea that tomorrow at half past seven o'clock a monstrous, unsuspected event will suddenly take place; that on Thursday next a complete revolution will be accomplished at a single blow, that a revelation, a redemption, the advent of a new age is imminent—this is frequently observed among the insane, it is a mystic delirium" (Nordau, 544). Nordau often outdid his master; indeed, Lombroso found it necessary, in the sixth edition of *Genio e degenerazione,* to chastise him severely for overzealous interpretations and applications of the master's theories. But on this point there is no dissent. In *Gli anarchici,* Lombroso discredits the aims of the Paris Commune by pointing out, "Se, fatta qualche rara eccezione, alcuno si sollevò, furono gli spostati, i criminali, i pazzi, gli alcoolisti" (69) ["If anyone rose up, with rare exceptions they were the misfits, criminals, madmen, and alcoholics"]. In his studies of genius, of criminals and anarchists, Lombroso employs

of anarchism draws freely from other revolutionary discourses. The distinguishing feature of anarchism, for Lombroso, is its "prematurity": "E qui appare la distinzione fra le rivoluzioni propriamente dette che sono un effetto lento, preparato, necessario, tutt'al più precipitato da qualche genio nevrotico o da qualche accidente storico, e le rivolte o sedizioni, frutti di un'incubazione artificiale a temperatura esagerata, di embrioni predestinati a morire. La rivoluzione è l'espressione storica dell'evoluzione, calma, ma estesa e sicura. . . . Questa non è dunque una malattia, ma una fase necessaria dello sviluppo della specie. Le sedizioni invece sono opera di pochi, corrispondono a cause poco importanti, sovente locali o personali, frequenti presso i popoli poco civili, come a San Domingo. . . . i delinquenti e i pazzi vi partecipano in maggior copia spintivi dalla loro morbosità a pensare, a sentire diversamente dagli onesti e sani" ["And here emerges the distinction between what are properly called revolutions, which are a slow, prepared, and necessary effect, at the most precipitated by some neurotic genius or by historical accident, and revolts or seditions, which are the fruit of an artificial incubation at an exaggerated temperature and of embryos predestined to die. Revolution is the historical expression of evolution, calm but wide-ranging and sure. . . . This, then, is not a sickness but a necessary phase in the development of the species. Seditions instead are the work of a few, they correspond to causes of little importance, often of a local or personal nature, frequent in uncivilized peoples, as in San Domingo. . . . criminals and madmen participate in them in greater numbers, urged on by their sickliness to think and feel differently from the healthy and honest"]. Cesare Lombroso, *Gli anarchici* (1894; rpt. Rome: Napoleone, 1972), 56–57, hereafter cited in the text.

a sort of magnified metalepsis whereby groups that have appeared most recently (decadent artists, political activists, urban criminals) are described as atavistic and archaic rather than, as in Marxist discourse, the products of modern industrialization. Degenerates, those who preserve characteristics of an earlier evolutionary stage, are in fact those newly generated in nineteenth-century cities. Lombroso's rhetoric of sickness removes these undesirables and relegates contemporary history to prehistory. For both Marxist literary criticism and the discourse on sickness, the decadents are political antagonists: for the former, they represent bourgeois decadence and thus are too far to the right; for the latter, they are too far to the left, criminal and even subhuman. The marriage of the two only thickens the screen, the blackened layer that obscures our view of decadent texts.

The deep distrust of the figurality of language which informs the notion that rhetoric is nothing but a grab bag of linguistic baubles, figures that disfigure thought, prevents another Marxist critic, Antonio Gramsci, from reading the decadents. Indeed, it makes reading itself difficult if not impossible, especially when the texts involved trace their genealogies to statements like Baudelaire's "éloge du maquillage" and to symbolist poetry. "D'Annunzio," writes Gramsci, "è stato l'ultimo accesso di malattia del popolo italiano" ["D'Annunzio was the Italian people's last bout of illness"].[13] One might expect this illness to be *fascismo* or *superuomismo*. But no, the malady D'Annunzio communicated to Italians is none other than style, and the awareness that language is not a transparent neutral vehicle for the transmission of thought. Rhetoric, in this rhetoric of antirhetoric, is sick.[14] "La sobrietà, la semplicità, l'immediatezza" ["The sobriety, the simplicity, the immediacy"] that should characterize "spontaneous" expression become unrecognizable when pockmarked by "l'ipocrisia stilistica" ["stylistic hypocrisy"]. Led by this reasoning to apologetically reaffirm a distinction between form and content, Gramsci claims that those writers who emphasize content are more democratic while those who

13. Antonio Gramsci, *Letteratura e vita nazionale,* ed. Valentino Gerratana, Istituto Gramsci (Rome: Riuniti, 1977), 71.

14. See Paolo Valesio's discussion of the rhetoric of antirhetoric in *Novantiqua* (Bloomington: Indiana University Press, 1982), 41–60.

chiacchierano di forma, ecc. contro il contenuto, sono com-
pletamente vuoti, accozzano parole che non sempre si tengono
neanche secondo grammatica (esempio Ungaretti); per tec-
nica, forma ecc. intendono vacuità di gergo da conventicola
di teste vuote.[15]

[chatter on about form, etc., against content are completely
empty; they throw together words that don't hold even according to grammar (Ungaretti is an example). By technique,
form, etc., they mean the vacuousness of the jargon of an
empty-headed clique.]

D'Annunzio and his dishonest clique hide an intellectual vacuum
behind their swollen, bombastic rhetoric; plain, simple speech lives
instead on the island of health. Croce, less an adversary than
Gramsci admits and certainly more sensitive to poetic resonance,
nods in assent: Gabriele D'Annunzio, Giovanni Pascoli, and Antonio Fogazzaro labor together in "la grande industria del vuoto"
["the great industry of the void"].[16]
    Is an embarrassment of stylistic riches a cosmetic for intellectual
poverty? Max Nordau spares no rhetorical riches in voicing his
agreement. Let us look at the portrait of Verlaine that hangs in his
gallery of the pathological:

We see a repulsive degenerate subject with asymmetric skull
and Mongolian face, an impulsive vagabond and dipsomaniac,
who, under the most disgraceful circumstances, was placed in
gaol; an emotional dreamer of feeble intellect, who painfully
fights against his bad impulses, and in his misery often utters
touching notes of complaint; a mystic whose qualmish consciousness is flooded with ideas of God and saints, and a dotard
who manifests the absence of any definite thought in his mind
by incoherent speech, meaningless expressions and motley images. In lunatic asylums there are many patients whose disease
is less deep-seated and incurable than is that of this irresponsible

15. Gramsci, 71–72.
16. Benedetto Croce, "Di un carattere della più recente letteratura italiana,"
in La letteratura della nuova Italia (Bari: Laterza, 1915), 4:186.

circulaire at large, whom only ignorant judges would have condemned for his epileptoid crimes. (Nordau, 128)

Nordau offers a medical definition of the term *circulaire:* "This not
very happy expression, invented by French psychiatry, denotes that
form of mental disease in which states of excitement and depression
follow each other in regular succession. The period of excitement
coincides with the irresistible impulses to misdeeds and blasphemous language; that of dejection with the paroxysms of contrition
and piety. The *circulaires* belong to the worst species of the
degenerate. . . . The *circulaires* are, by the nature of their affliction,
condemned to be vagabonds or thieves, unless they belong to
rich families. . . . [Verlaine] has loafed about all the highways of
France" (Nordau, 123). French psychiatry may have invented the
term *circulaire,* but in doing so its practitioners did not invent the
decadent phenomenon to which it refers, nor does the new term
completely mask the "original" one, the flaneur. Lombroso had
identified facial and cranial dissymmetries as stigmata of degeneration, to be found in criminals and geniuses alike. They are accompanied by other symptoms: limitation of the visual field (strange
measure of artistic vision!), hypertrophy of facial features and various organs, atrophy of other characteristics, cellular disintegration,
alcoholism, epilepsy, hysteria, and a generalized sensory obtuseness
to which Nordau attributes the synaesthetic phenomenon whereby
Baudelaire "saw with the nose" (Nordau, 296). Impressionist painters similarly suffered from "nystagmus, or trembling of the eyeball"
(Nordau, 27), due to hysterical contraction of the retina. Lombroso
had also specified certain peculiarities of linguistic practice, found
especially in "graphomaniacs," as degenerative symptoms: "l'inter-
pretazione mistica dei fatti più semplici, l'abuso dei simboli, delle
parole speciali che diventano a volte il modo esclusivo d'esprimersi"
["the mystical interpretation of the most simple facts, the abuse of
symbols and of special words that at times become the only means
of expression"].[17] The islanders of normalcy observe a pathological
other, tyrannized by physiology; to this other is transferred any
and all aberrant sexuality (woman, already the Other, is *ab ovo*

17. Cesare Lombroso, *L'uomo di genio in rapporto alla psichiatria, alla storia ed
all'estetica,* 6th ed. (Turin: Fratelli Bocca, 1894), 7, hereafter cited in the text.

degenerate). Paul Verlaine, then, is just what the doctor ordered: his poetic style and his style of life perfectly fit the degenerate nosology. Symbolist poetry merely confirms Nordau's diagnosis of this asymmetrical "Mongolian." I quote at length to let the "average" speak:

> The Symbolists, so far as they are honestly degenerate and imbecile, can think only in a mystical, i.e., in a confused way. The unknown is to them more powerful than the known; the activity of the organic nerves preponderates over that of the cerebral cortex; their emotions overrule their ideas. When persons of this kind have poetic and artistic instincts, they naturally want to give expression to their own mental state. They cannot make use of definite words of clear import, for their own consciousness holds no clearly-defined univocal ideas which could be embodied in such words. They choose, therefore, vague equivocal words, because these best conform to their ambiguous and equivocal ideas. . . . Clear speech serves the purpose of communication of the actual. It has, therefore, no value in the eyes of a degenerate subject. (Nordau, 118).

Nordau is perhaps not so "stupid" as he might seem, in much the same way as the readers of the Inquisition were remarkably shrewd in identifying texts that might be poison for popular consumption. Decadents were *not* interested in clear speech and "the communication of the actual." He listens, at stethoscope's length, to Verlaine's poetry: "The second peculiarity of Verlaine's style is the other mark of mental debility, viz. the combination of completely disconnected nouns and adjectives, which suggest each other, either through a senseless meandering by way of associated ideas, or through a similarity of sound" (Nordau, 126).

This stylistic appreciation leads us back to Gramsci, having learned through our detour that decadents do have ideas: ambiguous and equivocal ones. "Rhetoric" in Gramsci's discourse is a translucent screen through which we glimpse the shadowy presence of a repression. That which is ideologically unacceptable does not exist as thought but "merely" as rhetoric, as jargon, as "senseless meandering." Negation of the very existence of "decadent ideas" stems from a repudiation of the validity of those ideas: Nordau the positivist cannot admit the possibility of a mystic mode of thought (and "mystic," you will remember, has as at least one of its interpretants "revolutionary"); he retranslates the word, hurriedly reducing it to "confused." Gramsci's denial is perhaps more ambiguous; D'Annunzian sickness has already been cured by journalistic prose, but the cure has rendered the patient perhaps too healthy:

> Però l'ha impoverita e stremenzita e anche questo è un danno. . . . Nè si dica che di tale quistione non occorre occuparsi: anzi, la formazione di una prosa vivace ed espressiva e nello stesso tempo sobria e misurata deve essere uno dei fini culturali da proporsi.[18]

> [Yet it [journalistic practice] has impoverished and stunted it [prose] and this, too, is harmful. . . . And let no one say that one should not worry about this problem: on the contrary, the formation of a lively and expressive prose that would at the same time be sober and measured must be one of the cultural goals that we set for ourselves.]

An ideal prose, at once lively and sober. Is there not perhaps a touch of *ressentiment* in this disdain of D'Annunzio by a man who, as Pasolini sacrilegiously and courageously pointed out, did not write well?[19] In the context of the Italian critical tradition, such a suspicion is not merely a belletristic smear tactic but a truly political problem. Indeed, Italian critics find themselves in some-

---

18. Gramsci, 72–73.

19. See Pier Paolo Pasolini, "Due righe sulla lingua di Gramsci," in *Le belle bandiere* (Rome: Riuniti, 1977). This essay first appeared in 1965 in Pasolini's weekly column in *Vie Nuove,* and anticipated the elaborated version, "Laboratorio I: Appunti en poète per una linguistica marxista; II, La sceneggiatura come struttura che vuol essere altre strutture," in *Nuovi Argomenti,* n.s. 1 (January–March 1966): 14–54. Pasolini describes the young Gramsci's Italian as "bad" (*Nuovi Argomenti,* 14) and "impossible" (*Le belle bandiere,* 305) and points out that even after Gramsci's style seems to have matured, it is still marred by the sloppiness, political jargon, and manualistic blandness of his earlier style. An alternative or adversary must be invoked in defense of Gramsci, and that adversary is, not surprisingly, D'Annunzio or, more precisely, the D'Annunzian tradition, which represents, according to Pasolini, "aestheticizing authoritarianism" (*Nuovi Argomenti,* 17).

thing of a quandary over D'Annunzio's style. Paradigms of "good" and "bad" writing are, of course, ideologically conditioned, but by valorizing literary representations of the petite bourgeoisie (Luigi Pirandello, Federigo Tozzi, Italo Svevo) Italian criticism has honored as great writers authors who, as Giacomo Debenedetti has suggested, seem to be bad translators of beautiful books. "Good" writing is thus considered the vice of the right; "bad" writing, the virtue of the left. How, then, could the left write well? Is Gramsci perhaps forced to sever form from content in order to split the "bad" D'Annunzio (the unproblematized "Fascist" D'Annunzio) from the "good" D'Annunzio (who wrote "a lively and expressive prose"), to deny the existence of his ideas in order to make his prose an acceptable element in an ideal prose, to empty him of content in order to declare him vacuous? A touch of sickness makes health more visible.

In *The Case of Wagner,* Nietzsche himself exposes a bit of *ressentiment:* "Sickness itself can be a stimulant to life; only one has to be healthy enough for this stimulant." It is Nietzsche's text that we see *in filigrana* through the pages of Gramsci, Nietzsche's voice railing against Wagner that we hear: "Is Wagner a human being at all? Isn't he rather a sickness? He makes sick whatever he touches—*he has made music sick.*"[20] Its volume increased by the critical self-awareness of its tone, Nietzsche's voice drowns out Gramsci's. Nietzsche, the theorist of *ressentiment,* knew quite well when he himself exhibited it, when rancor upset his stomach. Wagner had been his sickness, Nietzsche writes; now he spits it back at Wagner, just as "slave morality" had spit back the epithet "evil" at the nobles who had labeled the slaves "bad." Wagner is a rival, a German (but not too German) rival. In the postscript to *The Case of Wagner,* Nietzsche adds as an "afterthought" on *Parsifal:* "I admire this work; I wish I had written it myself; failing that, I understand it."[21] Nietzsche's earlier admiration for Wagner turns into bilious criticism only when Nietzsche knows he has become Nietzsche and Wagner has, triumphantly, become Wagner: "My practice of war can be summed up in four propositions. First: I

---

20. Friedrich Nietzsche, *The Case of Wagner,* ed. and trans. Walter Kaufmann (New York: Vintage Books, 1967), 164, 165.
21. Ibid., 184.

only attack causes that are victorious. . . . Thus I attacked Wagner—more precisely, the falseness, the half-couth instincts of our 'culture' which mistakes the subtle for the rich, and the late for the great."[22] The two have become worthy of rivalry not only because the cause attacked has become victorious (for Wagner, the elder, had been "victorious" for some time), but also because the attacker feels sure of his own victory. If Wagner "gives his name to the ruin of music," then Nietzsche gives his to the "ruin" of philosophy, to the death of philosophy as metaphysics and to its rebirth as literature. It is when philosophy becomes poetry that Nietzsche perceives Wagner as an artistic rival. Energized by an ulcerous anxiety of influence, Nietzsche adds two postscripts and an epilogue to *The Case of Wagner* and later gathers other drops of venom in *Nietzsche contra Wagner* as a further antidote to his youthful sickness.

Gramsci was perhaps not healthy enough to absorb the D'Annunzian stylistic germ, but Benedetto Croce allowed himself to be contaminated. D'Annunzio is for Croce, in some though not all ways, what Wagner was for Nietzsche—an ever-present figure in his writing, an object of both admiration and vituperation: "Egli non ha avuto quel che si dice evoluzione o progresso, ma un mutare apparente e un persistere reale" ["He did not have what one calls evolution or progress, but rather an apparent change and a real persistence"].[23] Benedetto Croce's description of D'Annunzio's nondevelopment perhaps better describes the nondevelopment of anti-D'Annunzian criticism. The ideologeme of D'Annunzian sickness is passed on from Croce and G. A. Borgese to Gramsci and his *nipotini,* Carlo Salinari and Arcangelo Leone de Castris, like a package unexamined by tired customs officers too intent upon sequestering other forbidden Crocean goods. Apparent change but real persistence—each time we return to our task of unpacking we discover a new element in examining the "same" object. Another facet of the "sickness" of rhetoric, of D'Annunzio's prose style, is angled into visibility as we read Croce's analysis of D'Annunzio,

22. Nietzsche, *Ecce Homo,* ed. and trans. Walter Kaufmann (New York: Vintage Books, 1967), 232.

23. Benedetto Croce, "Gabriele D'Annunzio," in *La letteratura della nuova Italia* (Bari: Laterza, 1915), 4:24.

Pascoli, and Fogazzaro, an antitrinity in Italian literature, a "trina bugia" ["triple lie"] opposed to the true Carduccian faith: "Nel passare da Giosuè Carducci, a questi tre, sembra, a volte, come di passare da un uomo sano a tre ammalati di nervi" ["In passing from Giosuè Carducci to these three, it seems at times as though we were passing from a healthy man to three neurotics"].[24] In the 1907 essay "Di un carattere della più recente letteratura italiana" ["On a characteristic of the most recent Italian literature"], Croce defined this sickness as spiritual emptiness and, once again, insincerity, an emptiness created by the absence of Carduccian ideals—heroism, love, country, family, glory, death, and "la virile malinconia" ["virile melancholy"]. That D'Annunzio's representation of love is not wholesome enough but violent and sadistic, Croce tells us; that his patriotic ideas are not nationalistic but rather too imperialistic, Croce tells us; that D'Annunzian babies are merely "complessi di cellule che si contraggono o esseri malati o deformi" ["complexes of cells that contract or sick or deformed beings"] and that incestuous titillation does not become the ideal family, Croce tells us that, too. But virile? Would it not seem that D'Annunzio's preoccupation (according to Croce and Croceans alike) with sensuality and voluptuousness, with cruelty and sadism, were at least virile? Does Croce not tell us that Tullio Hermil, protagonist of *L'Innocente,* is motivated by "tormentose visioni falliche" ["tormenting phallic visions"], which, it is implied, also plague the author? Or is it perhaps Croce who is tormented by such visions? Certainly "virile melancholy" seems to be not a Carduccian ideal so much as a stylistic description, and a stylistic description that we find once again in *La storia d'Italia dal 1871 al 1915,* when Croce dismembers the body of D'Annunzio's work in order to repackage it for posterity.

In questa cerchia, egli era artista splendidissimo, e talune delle liriche del *Canto Novo* e della *Chimera,* e molte pagine

24. Croce, "Di un carattere della più recente letteratura italiana," in *La letteratura della nuova Italia* (Bari: Laterza, 1929), 4:199. In this third edition, revised by the author, "tre ammalati di nervi" replaces the earlier, more Lombrosian term "tre neurastenici," which appears in the same context in the 1915 edition.

del *Trionfo della Morte* e di altri romanzi, certe scene della *Figlia di Iorio* e le maggiori liriche del libro di *Alcione* saranno ricordate nella storia della poesia, se non della grande poesia italiana: ché, per la grande, a lui mancava la pienezza di umanità, la virilità carducciana o foscoliana.[25]

[In this circle, he was a most splendid artist, and some of the lyrics of the *Canto novo* and of the *Chimera,* and many pages of *The Triumph of Death* and of other novels, certain scenes of *The Daughter of Iorio* and the major lyrics of *Alcione* will be remembered in the history of poetry, if not that of great Italian poetry, for he lacked the fullness of humanity, the virility of a Carducci or a Foscolo necessary for greatness.]

Though lacking in fullness and virility, D'Annunzio had "gonfiato e falsato alcune sue brevi ispirazioni" ["swollen and falsified some of his brief inspirations"]; in D'Annunzio's style, in his very titles, there is "un certo che di gonfio e di sproporzionato" ["something swollen and out of proportion"]. "Stile gonfio" is a syntagm usually translated as "bombastic style," yet Croce himself (and even more so, Borgese) gives us reason to hear the literal "swollen, turgid" beneath the transferred meaning. Turgidity of style alternates with *fiacchezza,* "limpness," and sterility; clarity and simplicity of style are replaced by tumid images that deflate upon examination ("ampie volute di frasi immaginifiche, che parevano dire grandi cose, e sfumavano nel vago, illudendo e deludendo" ["ample spirals of imaginific sentences that seemed to say great things, and vanished into the haze, deluding and disappointing"]).[26] Rhetorical richness not only falsifies but is also a symptom of eviration. Or is an objection to D'Annunzio's fuller exploration of eros, and to the feminization of the male protagonist thematized in decadent narrative, here projected into a stylistic analysis? An image of a D'Annunzio exhausted by orgies appears in both Croce and Borgese, but such an orgiastic image has perhaps less to do with his writings than with critics titillated by anecdotes of the author's life.

25. Croce, *La storia d'Italia dal 1871 al 1915,* 5th ed. (1927; Bari: Laterza, 1934), 166.
26. Ibid., 50, 51, 260.

G. A. Borgese, in *Gabriele D'Annunzio,* reads the life through the works, the spiritual condition of the author as a first period of sensual and sexual vigor followed by "una languida voluttà nella contemplazione della propria fiacchezza" ["a languid voluptuousness in the contemplation of his own limpness"]. The fourth and following chapters of his monograph are devoted to an analysis of "la malattia dannunziana" ["the D'Annunzian sickness"], of the "bad" D'Annunzio (here, once again, the good D'Annunzio is split from the bad). The D'Annunzian malady seems to be hereditary; it joins a long line of -isms (or is it -itises?): Boccaccism, Petrarchism, Arcadism—which in turn stem from Ciceronian rhetoric ("Cicerone fu, in tutte le malattie della letteratura italiana . . . il modello della prosa" ["Cicero was the model of prose . . . of all illnesses of Italian literature"]).[27] The D'Annunzian illness is further aggravated by injections of Wagner and Venetian painting. But the real objection is to the poeticization of prose, to what is perceived as a surfeit of signifiers that conceal a poverty of the signified, of syllables that "esasperano anche fuor di proposito il significato" ["irrelevantly exasperate the meaning"], an abuse of superlatives and adjectives.

A questo modo il suo stile diventa gonfio e lungagginoso; e quel suo periodo, che a prima vista sembra un miracolo di dirittura, di logica e di forza, considerato più da vicino si rivela troppo spesso per una pinguedine inerte, scarsa di giunture e d'ossa, incapace di reggersi in piedi e studiosamente arrotondata in una floridezza molle, che tappa tutti i buchi e biancheggia di uno splendore che non è forza nè luce. Manca di snellezza, di asciuttezza, di rapidità. E vedendolo così prospero, ed impettito per la mal celata difficoltà che ha di procedere e di muoversi, voi desiderate qualche volta il fervido anacoluto di Cellini, il ritmo zoppicante di Machiavelli, la durezza granitica di Alfieri, la bonomia quasi sciatta di Manzoni, la magrezza sanguigna di Leopardi.[28]

27. G. A. Borgese, *Gabriele D'Annunzio* (1909; rpt. Milan: Bompiani, 1932), 66, 193.
28. Ibid., 187. "Stile gonfio" appears only in the 1932 edition; in the 1909 and 1951 editions, we find "stile tronfio" in its place.

[In this way his style becomes swollen and long-winded, and that sentence of his, which at first seems a miracle of rectitude, of logic and strength, when considered at closer range too often reveals itself to be an inert fattiness with few joints and bones, incapable of standing on its own and deliberately rounded out in a soft rosy glow that stops up all the holes and glows white in a splendor that is neither strength nor light. It lacks slenderness, dryness, rapidity. And seeing it so prosperous and stiff on account of the poorly concealed difficulty that it has in proceeding and moving along, you sometimes desire Cellini's fervid anacoluthon, Machiavelli's limping rhythm, Alfieri's granitelike hardness, Manzoni's almost careless good humor, Leopardi's sanguine slenderness.]

Style, at first tumid and a miracle of rectitude, recoils at the critic's touch and becomes inert fleshiness deprived of rigidifying bone. A soft rosy glow whitens and "stops up all the holes." Yet the critic's desire remains unfulfilled; immediately the image of erection (*impettito*) is recalled, an erectness incapable of movement (because all the holes are blocked?), and desire is displaced to the granitelike hardness of Alfieri. "The question of style," writes Derrida, "is always the examination [examen], the weight of a pointed object."[29] D'Annunzio's style does not satisfy the critic; it is too soft, too round, too moist . . . almost too feminine. A promise unfulfilled, desire turns to the fervor of Cellini, to the rhythm of Machiavelli. Desire disappointed cloaks its disillusion in a diagnosis of sickness. Whiteness that is neither strength nor light is also whitewash. D'Annunzio's style is a whited sepulcher; the promise of sensual refinement is betrayed. Borgese continues:

Anche qui la malattia verbale non è che un sintomo dell'ispirazione malata. Come nell'ispirazione del D'Annunzio il crimine, la viltà, la libidine animale hanno aspetto di eroismo, così nel suo stile si drappeggiano di paludamenti grandiosi anche le cose più semplici. Come un certo tipo di bel tiranno

29. Jacques Derrida, *Spurs: Nietzsche's Styles/Eperons: Les styles de Nietzsche,* trans. Barbara Harlow (Chicago: University of Chicago Press, 1979), 37, trans. modified.

o una certa immaginazione sadico-guerresca domina con la fissità di una mania il suo cervello, così un certo ideale determinato di periodo e di verso tronca il respiro alla libertà del suo stile.[30]

[Here, too, the verbal sickness is nothing other than a symptom of sick inspiration. Just as crime, cowardice, and animal lust take on the appearance of heroism in D'Annunzio's inspiration, so in his style even the simplest things are draped in grandiose paludaments. Just as a certain kind of beautiful tyrant or a certain sadistic-warlike imagination dominates his brain with the fixity of a mania, so a certain ideal of sentence and verse cuts short his style's aspiration to freedom.]

What is "low" is disguised and elevated by a turgid style; what seems to be an upright style is instead feminine softness. If sadism dominates the author's imagination (something that remains to be explored), there is at least a hint of longing for a *bel tiranno* in the critic. It is not eros as a poetic concern which disturbs Croce and Borgese but the sort of eros D'Annunzio seems both to depict and to personify, an eros at once too high and too low, too powerful and too languid, expressed in a style seemingly too virile and yet somehow too feminine. Accepting D'Annunzio's own paronomastic motto, *Erotica/Heroica,* they interpolate the missing third term, *Retorica,* and transfer to it their objections to any other term in the triad.

From the Lombrosian island of normalcy, the view of genius includes sterility as an important degenerative feature, complemented by various forms of aberrant sexuality: "La natura ha, come gli uomini, orrore del genio e sterilizza (vedasi anche qui un'altra analogia del genio con l'ingegno) quegli animali che osano pensare qualche poco di più dei loro compagni di specie" ["Like men, nature abominates and sterilizes (note here another analogy of genius to brilliance) those animals who dare to think a little more than their fellow members of the species"].[31] Hypertrophy of any organ must be accompanied by atrophy of another; an overdevel-

30. Borgese, 188.
31. Lombroso, *Genio e degenerazione* (Palermo: Remo Sandron, 1897), 258.

oped intellect provokes nature into abolishing fecundity. Sterility does not, however, imply the absence of sexual activity but rather its unrestrained and irregular development. Lombroso's theory, which so often relies upon anecdote, photographs, quotations from Balzac or Stendhal rather than upon an explanatory model, here finds confirmation in a list of "genii alienati" ["alienated geniuses"]:

> Quasi tutti, poi, questi grandi, presentarono anche anomalie nelle funzioni riproduttrici. Tasso fu di esagerata libidine nella giovinezza, di rigida castità dopo i trentotto anni; viceversa Cardano, impotente da giovane, a trentacinque si fa libidinosissimo. —Pascal, sensuale nella prima gioventù, più tardi crede fin delittuoso il bacio materno. —Rousseau era affetto da ipospadia e spermatorrea, e, come Baudelaire, Cesare, Winkelmann [*sic*], Cellini, Michelangelo e molti altri, aveva una perversione sessuale. (*L'uomo di genio*, 536)

> [Almost all of these great men exhibited anomalies in their reproductive functions. Tasso possessed exaggerated lust in his youth, rigid chastity after the age of thirty-eight. Cardano was precisely the opposite: impotent as a youth, at the age of thirty-five he became extremely lustful. Sensual in his early youth, Pascal later thought even his mother's kiss was criminal. Rousseau was afflicted by hypospadia and spermatorrhea, and like Baudelaire, Caesar, Winckelmann, Cellini, Michelangelo, and many others, had a sexual perversion.]

"Genius" is a sort of dinosaur, so top-heavy that it can no longer reproduce itself, too overspecialized in the struggle for survival, where mediocrity wins out. Its sexuality follows the paths of perversion. Genius represents both the highest evolutionary development and the most atavistic throwback, for sterility appears in the lowest animals as intelligence grows. As organisms specialize, sexual differentiation is blurred. Lombroso addresses the problem as it appears in bees, ants, and termites:

> Ora queste tre specie d'animali sono le sole nella natura . . . che offrano una sterilità completa negli individui che lavorano, sì che costituiscono una specie a parte nelle stesse famiglie, di

femmine assolutamente sterili con organi nervosi ipertrofici e sessuali atrofici—che si chiamano neutri; mentre i veri maschi e le vere femmine, che conservano l'attività sessuale, non mostrano traccia di maggiore intelligenza. (*L'uomo di genio,* 623)

[Now these three animal species are the only ones in nature . . . that exhibit complete sterility in the individuals who work, such that they constitute in their own families a separate species of absolutely sterile females with hypertrophic nervous organs and atrophic sexual organs. These are called neuters. The true males and females, who retain sexual activity, do not show traces of greater intelligence.]

This sudden appearance of ants, bees, and termites may jar the reader, but Lombroso takes the term *atavism* seriously; his chapter "L'atavismo del genio" ["The atavism of genius"] relies on just such zoological scenarios. In this "lower" example, we may read more clearly what is implied by the "higher" one—that sterility is a front for the confusion of sexual difference. The highest development is a neuter(ed) being, a being in whom high and low, masculine and feminine are inseparable. Advanced human development takes place in the male rather than the female, however, for the human female is several rungs down, arrested in her upward climb: "Anche nella scala zoologica le specie più basse si sviluppano più precocemente di quelle d'ordine più elevato: e la donna è più precoce dell'uomo" (*L'uomo di genio,* 625) ["On the zoological ladder as well, the lower species develop more precociously than higher orders; and woman is more precocious than man"]. Lombroso is a pre-Freudian, yes, but he shares with Freud the conclusion that a woman is but an undeveloped man. Yet this blurring of difference is not utopian, it does not represent a longed-for androgyny, nor is it the appearance of a Jungian anima in an artistic temperament. What Freud theorizes in individual ontogeny, Lombroso explains through phylogeny: in the amoebic beginning, there was no sexual difference, only a sort of polymorphic perversity. The degenerative return of nondifference is not utopian but criminal.

Lombroso, unlike Nordau, describes sexual aberration in genius with equanimity; his study of genius is colored by admiration for, and self-identification with, greatness and artistic achievement, no matter how degenerate. It is rather in his monumental study, *La donna delinquente, la prostituta e la donna normale,* that we discover criminality in the abolition of difference. Genius had been an entirely masculine phenomenon, for as Lombroso affirmed in *L'uomo di genio,*

> E quando la genialità compare nella donna è sempre associata a grandi anomalie: e la più grande è la somiglianza coi maschi—la virilità. Goncourt aveva scritto giustamente: "Il n'y a pas de femmes de génie: lorsqu'elles sont des génies, elles sonts des hommes." (261)

> [And when genius appears in woman it is always associated with great anomalies, the greatest of which is their resemblance to males: virility. Goncourt wrote correctly: "There are no women genuises; when women are geniuses, they are men."]

In *La donna delinquente* it becomes clear that even the normal woman has but a precarious existence. Normal femininity must be a perfect mirror-negative of masculinity, a negative mirror image rarely discovered. Lombroso searches for such a face in his readings of the *visages moralisés* that he describes, reproduces in photographs, measures with craniometers, *visages moralisés* that appear along a continuum from amoebas which have no distinct sex or have both, to the human range of masculine and feminine. The slippage between the two causes delirium, and his science grips a grid of control—of numbers, of statistics presented without interpretative keys or scales—laid upon an indistinct flow of characteristics. The scientist himself despairs, and he admits how rickety is his grid:

> Quando trent'anni fa, uno di noi iniziò questi studi, giurava sull'antropometria, specie cranica, applicata allo studio di delinquenti; vi vedeva la tavola di salvezza contro la metafisica, l'apriorismo dominante in tutti gli studi che toccavano dell'uomo. . . . Ma, come accade delle cose umane, l'uso degenerando in abuso, mi mostrò la vanità delle mie speranze, il danno, anzi, enorme della troppa fiducia. Tutta la discrepanza, infatti, dei moderni anche più ponderati antropologi,

che non sono, infine, che antropometri, contro noi, dipende appunto da questo che le differenze in misure dall'anormale al normale sono così poche che, salvo una delicatissima ricerca, non si rinvengono. . . . Ma non però quelle misure devonsi abbandonare, non fosse altro come cornice del quadro, come simbolo, come bandiera di una scuola che fa della cifra la migliore sua arma.[32]

[When, thirty years ago, one of us began this research, he swore by anthropometry, especially cranial, applied to the study of criminals. He saw in anthropometry its salvation from meta-physics, from the a priorism dominant in all the fields that dealt with man. . . . But as is the way with all things human, as use degenerated into abuse I saw the vanity of my hopes, indeed the enormous harm of excessive faith. In fact, all of the disagree-ment between us and even the most cautious modern anthropol-ogists, who are finally merely anthropometrists, depends on the fact that the differences in measurements between the abnormal and the normal are so small that they do not even appear except in the most delicate research. . . . And yet those measurements must not be abandoned, even if only as the picture frame, as a symbol, as the banner of a school that makes the number/cipher its best weapon.]

Such a painful admission appears in none of the other, frequently revised and republished studies, *L'uomo delinquente, Gli anarchici, L'uomo di genio, Genio e degenerazione,* though the same methods and physiognomic measures are adopted for them all.[33] The drawings

---

32. Lombroso and G. Ferrero, *La donna delinquente, la prostituta e la donna normale* (Turin: L. Roux, 1893), 261–62, hereafter cited in the text.

33. The desperately empirical register of physiological description employed in all Lombroso's studies is supplemented in *La donna delinquente* by a greater quantity of nonempirical material and commentary. The folklore, proverbs, and literary representations included in that study are symptomatic of a *mentalité* more resistant to the will to "scientific" observation. While the literary references included in *L'uomo di genio* and *Genio e degenerazione* are often taken from the "patient's" writings, such evidence is presumably unavailable when dealing with women, because of "quella inferiorità nei centri grafici che notammo anche nella donna normale" ["that inferiority in the graphic centers which we noted in the normal woman as well"] (464). Deprived of a means of self-representation,

of the skulls of Ugo Foscolo and Immanuel Kant, the photographs of Russian prostitutes and Wagner, the measurements of Hottentot hymens—all remain as symbols but no longer as scientific evidence. They remain as icons of a lost positivistic faith. Is it the search for the *visage* of normal femininity that leads Lombroso to despair of the "cifra," a femininity that is itself a cipher? He does find the virile woman of genius, the virile female criminal, the virile prostitute, but feminine normalcy seems an impossibility. Female virility returns as a refrain to every category examined. Of prostitutes: "Ora le nostre ree si avvicinano più alle femmine antiche e ancor più ai maschi antichi" (*La donna,* 280) ["Now our female criminals are closer to ancient females and closer yet to ancient males"]. Of born criminals: "Tale è in complesso la fisonomia morale della criminale nata che mostra cioè una tendenza fortissima a confondersi col tipo maschile" (*La donna,* 467) ["Such is, on the whole, the moral physiognomy of the born female criminal, who exhibits a very strong tendency to be confused with the male type"]. And of common criminals: "Quello che sopratutto colpisce è la virilità; sono tipi (e qualche volta vestiari) di maschio grossolano sopra corpi di femmina" (*La donna,* 342) ["What is most striking is their virility: they are crude masculine types, and sometimes masculine clothing, on female bodies"]. Crude masculinity that dresses a female body, a seemingly virile style that conceals a languid softness—Lombroso's description of the degenerate woman is not far from Borgese's analysis of a sort of decadent literary transvestitism.

My intention is not to "lower" Borgese's stylistic description to Lombroso's evolutionary delirium or to "elevate" Lombroso's criminological meditation to the level of sophisticated literary criticism. On the contrary, I mean to "average" them, apart from questions of cultural hierarchies, in order to uncover the coordinates of the antidecadent rhetoric of sickness. Croce and Borgese do not speak from a Jungian point of view of the reconciliation of opposites

woman can only be represented. Thus statistics from "scientific" experiments can appear alongside age-old commonplaces; the quantified results of a test of women's "ottusità dolorifica" ["obtuseness to pain"] are followed by the "conclusion": "Il fatto è anche notato dai proverbi: Li fimmini hannu setti spirdi comu li gatti / Le donne hanno l'anima attaccata con la colla cerviona" (61) ["The fact is also noted in proverbs: Females have seven souls like cats / Women have their souls attached with collagenous glue"].

or from a Freudian point of view (though they are contemporaries of Freud); instead, they object to con-fusion, to "femininity," and they recommend virility. Croce is more subtle because more literary than Lombroso, but the preoccupation persists. Both Croce, in *Storia d'Italia dal 1875 al 1915,* and Carlo Salinari, in *Miti e coscienza del decadentismo italiano,* recall the enchanted Circean gardens where the heroes of Ariosto's and Tasso's poems are waylaid as a figure for the confusion of masculine and feminine symptomatic of the D'Annunzian malady. A seductress enslaves the hero: Alcina, in *Orlando furioso,* enslaves Ruggiero in her "regno effeminato e molle" ["soft and effeminate realm"], stripping him of his warrior's strength. Tasso's Armida enchants Rinaldo and holds him until a fellow warrior offers Rinaldo a mirror-shield in which he observes his most unwarlike appearance, "dal troppo lusso effeminato" ["effeminated from too much luxury"].[34] Rinaldo and Ruggiero, however, free themselves of the bewitching siren songs and return to their virile pursuits; D'Annunzio, it would seem, remains garlanded and "molle," even when he becomes the D'Annunzio of political oratory. Croce writes, of the *Canzoni della gesta d'oltremare:*

> Quel che si avvertiva di sentito nelle nuove canzoni del D'Annunzio erano sempre le impressioni sensuali, soprattutto delle cose crudeli, turpi e ripugnanti, come fin dai primi suoi tentativi di uscire dai giardini di Alcina e affacciarsi agli spettacoli della patria e della guerra.[35]

> [What one felt were sincere in D'Annunzio's new poems were always sensual impressions, especially of cruel, foul, and repugnant things, as was the case since his first attempts to leave Alcina's gardens and face the spectacles of the fatherland and of war.]

That the gardens are recalled as a locus not only of sensuality but also of eviration becomes even clearer when Salinari takes up the

34. Ludovico Ariosto, *Orlando furioso,* ed. Lanfranco Caretti (Milan: Ricciardi, 1954), 7.48; Torquato Tasso, *Gerusalemme liberata,* ed. Lanfranco Caretti (Milan: Mondadori, 1979), 4.30.
   35. Croce, *La storia,* 277.

topos. The Marxist Salinari, whose introduction is predictably anti-Crocean, cannot but be aware that he cites Croce while citing Nietzsche, that, by referring to Armida rather than Alcina, he plays Tasso to Croce's Ariosto. Indeed, his study of decadentism is tailored to fit the Crocean paradigm: each of the three "ammalati di nervi" receives a chapter, and Pirandello replaces Carducci as sanity, as the "consciousness of the crisis." The Tassian Salinari, bound by ideological constraints, relies nonetheless upon the Ariostean Croce for the backbone of his tale:

> Dietro le danze e le risa di Zarathustra vi sono, dunque, questa stanchezza, questa tristezza, questi rimpianti. D'Annunzio, invece, si ferma nei giardini di Armida, non lascia dietro le cose belle: caso mai lascia innanzi la ricerca del vero e del certo. La sua stanchezza si deve al fatto che ha troppo goduto, la sua insoddisfazione (quando c'è) deriva dall'essersi fermato troppo e troppo spesso, di aver percorso poca strada sulla via dell'*idea*. Il dramma nicciano si capovolge, si svirilizza e s'immeschinisce.[36]

> [Behind Zarathustra's dances and laughter there are, then, this fatigue, this sadness, these regrets. D'Annunzio, instead, lingers in Armida's gardens; he does not leave behind the beautiful things. If anything, he leaves aside the search for the true and the certain. His fatigue is due to the fact that he has enjoyed too much, his dissatisfaction (when there is any) comes from having lingered too much and too often, from having made little progress on the road to the *idea*. The Nietzschean drama is overturned, evirated, made petty.]

The figure of Armida/Alcina is perhaps even stronger than the straightforward statement that D'Annunzio "evirates" Nietzsche and that this eviration is equivalent to a petty reading. This moment of fantasy (which dreams of another moment of fantasy) blooms as a symptom not only of an obsession with virility but of the powerful attraction D'Annunzio's siren song exerts upon the

36. Carlo Salinari, *Miti e coscienza del decadentismo italiano: D'Annunzio, Pascoli, Fogazzaro e Pirandello* (Milan: Feltrinelli, 1960), 81.

critic. Ah, to have enjoyed "too much," to have dallied, like D'Annunzio, "too long and too often!" One must stop one's ears to this siren song in order to continue along the path of the intellect to a more virile, warlike mode. D'Annunzio would have been "better" had he had the strength to abandon his "regno effeminato," Salinari tells us; yet even when he does venture away toward Nietzsche and toward political speeches, he continues to represent (for the critic) "effeminate sensuality." If Wagner was, for Nietzsche, a Midas who sickened all he touched, D'Annunzio is, for Croce and Salinari, a Midas who evirates all who come into contact with him. It is not surprising, then, to find yet another variation that figures D'Annunzio's texts themselves as sorceress, siren, and whore. Gian Pietro Lucini writes:

> Comunque, l'irrequieto viaggiatore ch'io era di quel tempo, in cerca di mia strada, che desiderava far altra, in ricognizione delle altrui virtù, che non desiderava imitare, piuttosto emulare, —e pur confuso e ben carezzato, nella mia ingenua giovanezza, dai suoni dell'Abruzzese, stregato, nelli occhi, dal suo lussuoso caleidoscopio, compiaciuto dal vanto della sua purezza, cui già si accostavano i professori delle scuole secondarie, maestri de' giornalisti d'oggidì; —comunque, anch'io diedi nella ragna tessami dai vezzi della allettatrice sua feminea prestanza. E non pensava ch'egli l'aveva messa in mostra di sulla finestra, come la Talanta aretinesca, allo zimbello e per uccellare, specialmente i più giovani ed i più alacri, per nutrir, poi, del meglio delle loro scarselle il suo mignone, ed era tanto arida di cuore, da reale cortigiana, come doveva essere per le necessità del suo mestiere, imbellettata il volto e contigiata di vesti, il tutto per eccitare, come la Babilonese biblica, alla lussuria, cioè alla idolatria.[37]

[The restless traveler that I was then, in search of his path and wanting to do something else, in recognition of others' virtues, did not wish to imitate but rather to emulate—and though confused and well caressed in my ingenuous youth by

---

37. Gian Pietro Lucini, *Antidannunziana* (Milan: Studio Editoriale Lombardo, 1914), 15.

the sounds of the Abruzzese, bewitched and bedazzled by his luxurious kaleidoscope, satisfied by the reputation of his purity, which high school teachers, the masters of today's journalists, were already accepting—I, too, fell into the web woven for me by the charms of his alluring feminine appearance. And that traveler that was I did not think that he had put it on display at the window, like Aretino's Talanta, as a decoy to catch the youngest and quickest, in order to nurture his darling with the best of their purses, and she was so hard-hearted like a true courtesan, as she had to be for her profession, with her face made up and adorned with robes, all to excite to lust and idolatry, like the biblical whore of Babylon.]

The text itself has become the sorceress's garden, and the critic, rather than D'Annunzio, bewitched. As in the Circean gardens of Armida and Alcina, the promise of satisfaction held out in the moment of enchantment is later deluded by an unveiling: the text is nothing but a painted whore. As we shall see, this "criticism" of D'Annunzio's texts is simply a repetition of their structure; Lucini is indeed caught in the web of the text.[38]

Lombroso, more secure upon his island, more confident of the "pathos of distance" which separates him from the pathological other, coolly describes the phenomenon already noted by the decadents themselves ("L'homme s'affine, se féminise, se divinise") and later troped by literary critics:

L'influenza della degenerazione tende sempre più a ravvicinare

38. In "Turning the Screw of Interpretation," Shoshana Felman lucidly describes how critics "act out" the texts that they presumably analyze: "The scene of the critical debate is thus a *repetition* of the scene dramatized in the text. The critical interpretation, in other words, not only elucidates the text but also reproduces it dramatically, unwittingly *participates in it.* Through its very reading, the text, so to speak, acts itself out. As a reading effect, this inadvertent 'acting out' is indeed uncanny: whichever way the reader turns, he can but be turned by the text, he can but *perform* it by *repeating* it." See *Literature and Psychoanalysis: The Question of Reading: Otherwise* (Baltimore: Johns Hopkins University Press, 1982), 101. The topos of the enchantress-turned-hag is discussed at greater length in Chapter 4.

e a confondere i due sessi, per cui si ha nei criminali l'infantilità
femminile nel maschio che lo mena alla pederastia, a cui
corrisponde la mascolinità delle donne, per una tendenza al
ritorno atavistico verso il periodo dell'ermafroditismo. La
prova ne è che in molte questa tendenza ha preceduto fino la
pubertà; che molte si compiacevano a vestirsi da maschio
. . . godevano a vedere organi femminili, sfuggivano i lavori
femminili. Difatti, secondo Schüle, nella pazzia morale e nella
epilessia, si riscontrano frequenti i casi di perversioni sessuali.
(*La donna,* 416)

[The influence of degeneration tends to confuse the two sexes
and bring them ever closer together. Hence one finds in male
criminals the female infantility that leads them to pederasty,
and in female criminals, a corresponding masculinity on account of a tendency to return atavistically to the period of
hermaphroditism. The proof of this is that in many women
this tendency even preceded puberty, and that many took
delight in dressing as males . . . enjoyed seeing the female
organs, and avoided feminine tasks. In fact, according to
Schüle, cases of sexual perversion are frequently associated
with moral madness and epilepsy.]

Epilepsy and "moral madness" are metonymies for genius; the
disease stands for the man; degeneration is also degenderation.
What was intended as a meditation on difference (healthy vs. sick,
pathological vs. normal, male vs. female, animal vs. human) ends
by recognizing similarity and reveals the impossibility of the project. Nature's upward evolutionary climb turns out to be a marching
in place. What the literary critics view with hostility, Lombroso
accepts with resignation and even optimism: there is no progress
without regress. Lombroso had, in the introduction to *La donna
delinquente,* warned the commonsensical reader that such contradic-
tion is part of the complex that the clear-eyed scientist must
discover and accept. And just as there is no progress without
regress, so there is no "genius," no literature, no music, no art, no
philosophy without sickness. For Lombroso, the healthy art(ist) of
Nordau or Croce or Lukács belongs to the realm of the counterna-

tural or, rather, cannot even be supposed to exist. He must, therefore, chastise his earnest disciple for grave misreading:

> M. Nordau, volendo esagerare un principio nuovo e giusto, quello di servirsi nella critica letteraria, più dell'esame personale degli autori che non delle loro opere, non ha però abbastanza distinto il mattoide, il quale non è se non un imbecille colla larva del genio, inetto ad ogni creazione, dal vero genio larvato di alienazione (paranoia in genere, monomania, epilessia), i cui prodotti erano, si può dire, di tanto più sublimi quanto più era il corpo malato, anzi perchè era malato; e allora avrebbe potuto accorgersi che il suo ostracismo colpiva tarquiniamente le più alte cime, da Wagner a Ibsen a Tolstoi, mentre lasciava intatte, perchè veramente meno ammalate, le creazioni mediocri. (*L'uomo di genio,* xii)

> [Max Nordau, in wanting to exaggerate a new and correct principle (that of utilizing more personal examination of the authors than of their works in literary criticism) has not, however, sufficiently distinguished the mattoid—who is nothing other than an imbecile with the outward sign of genius, inept at any creation—from the true genius marked by alienation (usually paranoia, monomania, epilepsy) whose products were, one might say, all the more sublime as the body was sicker, in fact, precisely because the body was sick. If he had distinguished between them, he would have realized that, in Tarquinian style, his ostracism struck down the highest peaks, from Wagner to Ibsen to Tolstoy, while it left intact mediocre creations because they were truly less sick.]

The island of normalcy has become a valley of mediocrity from which to observe with awe and respect the high peaks of sickness. There can be no generation without degeneration. Lombroso the positivist might be better described as a decadent positivist, for here he speaks the language of decadent writers, not the metalanguage of the critics, when he observes that sublimity is born of sickness. Anti-D'Annunzian criticism, instead, followed in the interpretive footsteps of Dr. Nordau. Lombroso shares in both. His texts occupy an important position in the genealogies of both the metalanguage

of anti-D'Annunzian critics and the language of D'Annunzio himself—a genealogical position, rather than that of "source" not
because sources cannot be traced but because the relationships
between these texts are fraught with all the tensions and disavowals,
desires and repressions that feed the family romance.[39] Despite
geographical, ideological, and generic differences, these texts all
participate in the decadent rhetoric of sickness and health, decay
and degeneration, pathology and normalcy.

The critics' antipathy for D'Annunzio fixes on erotic discourse
as a locus of pathology—either D'Annunzio's, or the critics', or
both. Lombroso's perhaps surprising sympathy for "sick genius"
suggests that we are dealing less with the representation of "period
illnesses" (on the order of the popular novel's fondness for tuberculo-
sis) or "illness as metaphor" than with a valorization of physiological
illness and alteration as the origin of psychic alterity. In order to
explore both suggestions, I leave behind the "bad air" of anti-
D'Annunzian criticism and move on not to fresh air but to the air
of the sickroom itself.

39. For a discussion of a genealogical approach to intertextuality, see Paolo
Valesio, "Genealogy of a Staged Scene: *Orlando furioso*, V," *Yale Italian Studies*
n.s. 1 (Spring 1980): 5–31.

[2] *The Scene of Convalescence*

The Horror of Origins

If the critics of decadent writers employ a Lombrosian rhetoric of sickness, the decadents themselves might be said to adopt a Baudelairean rhetoric of sickness in their descriptions of convalescence. Far from being terms of opprobrium, eviration and feminization of the (male) protagonist are constitutive elements of this rhetoric and of the decadent aesthetic. The critics' criticism is thus less an analysis of these texts than a repetition of the fundamental move whereby the decadents accepted their "negative" epithet and transformed it into praise. The critics, however, move in the opposite direction: they take the sickness, eviration, and feminization valorized by the decadents and transform those terms into defects and shortcomings.

The scenes of convalescence this chapter examines are four: Charles Baudelaire's *Peintre de la vie moderne,* J. K. Huysmans's *A rebours,* D'Annunzio's *Piacere,* and Friedrich Nietzsche's preface to the second edition of *The Gay Science.* The three names surrounding that of D'Annunzio represent obligatory citations in any study of decadence, citations made obligatory both by his critics and by D'Annunzio himself.[1] The problem posed by D'Annunzio's texts

1. Almost all the bibliography on D'Annunzio could be cited at this point; two articles covering this territory point out all the obligatory stops in a synthetic fashion: Giuseppe Petronio, "Il decadentismo: La parola e la cosa," and Norbert Jonard, "D'Annunzio romanziere decadente," both in *Quaderni del Vittoriale* 36 (1982): 9–48.

is not to uncover unacknowledged sources but to read and interpret an abundance of acknowledgments. The critic whose quest is for sources, in the traditional mode of source criticism, may well feel preempted by this abundance and find herself looking for depth when all is surface, for decadent texts flaunt their intertextuality, footnote themselves endlessly, self-consciously present their own literary genealogies. Indeed, a text such as *A rebours,* the so-called bible of decadence, might more aptly be termed the bibliography of decadence; it proposes not its own rereading for spiritual guidance but the reading of its sources for artistic guidance.² The predominance of metalanguage in *A rebours* represents a general tendency; the presence of metalanguage in fictional texts and of literary language in philosophical texts is a distinguishing feature of decadent narrative. Within the boundaries of individual texts (insofar as any text can be said to have boundaries) it is that metalanguage, that tension between language and metalanguage, which seems to bring all to the shimmering surface. Digging for buried sources in these texts is like searching for the vanishing point of a Gustav Klimt painting; in order to read either the literary text or the painting, a different perspective is needed.

A rebours is an extreme case, but *Il piacere,* too, is inlaid with intertextual references. Literary genealogies seem, in D'Annunzio's texts, to be traceable with ease, without anxiety, and critics have often followed these references as though they were the reassuring bread crumbs and pebbles strewn by Hansel and Gretel: the path to the good and true father. Thus the influences of Dostoevsky and Tolstoy can be noted in *L'Innocente,* of Nietzsche in *Trionfo della morte,* of Maupassant in *Le novelle della Pescara,* to name but a few.³

2. In the decadent code, literary guidance is spiritual guidance, just as spiritual guidance as well as sacred objects become literary objects. For an insightful investigation of how the language of decadent texts "metamorphoses" evangelical language, see Paolo Valesio, "Il coro degli Agrigentini," *Quaderni del Vittoriale* 36 (1982): 63–92.

3. Francesco Flora, in his *D'Annunzio* (Naples: Ricciardi, 1926), continues the list: "We have said it: in the final analysis, D'Annunzio's history would turn out to be a repetition of his sources, and the malicious would say, of his plagiarism. Queueing up we find Maupassant, Flaubert, Baudelaire, Zola, de Musset, Verlaine, Rimbaud, Péladan, Lorrain, Coppée, de Goncourt, de Banville, Gauthier, Maeterlinck, Verhaeren, de Régnier, Gide, France, Claudel: and then Tolstoy, Dostoevsky, and perhaps Korolenko; and Byron, Keats,

These clearly marked trails (the latter, one of the infamous *plagi*, is paradoxically the most clearly marked of all, the path so clear that D'Annunzio does not even bother to point to it) can be likened to the path of pebbles which, glowing in the moonlight, led the siblings safely home. In D'Annunzio's novels, those trails often lead to reassuring fathers who seem not to threaten the integrity of the text. The names of writers and poets, painters and musicians decorate D'Annunzio's texts as though they were paintings hung on the walls of a villa. In fact, D'Annunzio's last residence, Il Vittoriale degli Italiani, mirrors his texts and constitutes a metalanguage for his novels and poetry. It is a house of citation in which Dante's "Tre donne intorno al cor" is inscribed upon the beams of his bedroom; a jewel-encrusted tortoise like that of Huysmans's Jean Des Esseintes still sits on the dining table, and Michelangelo's Sibyls perch like bathing beauties above his bathtub. This easy quotation becomes, according to the notorious charges of plagiarism, sleazy quotation when D'Annunzio borrows freely from Maupassant, Verlaine, or Maeterlinck without paying "due homage." D'Annunzio seems to pose as the sort of figure Harold Bloom sees in Shakespeare: a strong father who absorbs his precursors absolutely.[4] For Bloom, however, D'Annunzio would come too

Shelley, Poe, Swinburne, Oscar Wilde, Kipling, Walt Whitman; and then Wagner, Nietzsche, and then Ibsen, and so forth. The list of Italian writers would be longer still, from Vettori to Megalotti to Tommaseo to Carducci, leaving aside the classics" (11). The classic accusations of plagiarism are Enrico Thovez, *Il pastore, il gregge e la zampogna* (Naples: Ricciardi, 1910), and *L'arco di Ulisse* (Naples: Ricciardi, 1921); and Gian Pietro Lucini, *Antidannunziana* (Milan: Studio Editoriale Lombardo, 1914).

4. "Shakespeare is the largest instance in the language of a phenomenon that stands outside the concern of this book: the absolute absorption of the precursor." Such absorption is possible only before the romantic watershed: "With the post-Enlightenment passion for Genius and the Sublime, there came anxiety too." Harold Bloom, *The Anxiety of Influence: A Theory of Poetry* (1973; rpt. London: Oxford University Press, 1981), 11, 27. If there is such anxiety in D'Annunzio's poetry, it is the absolute precursor in Italian poetry—Dante—who provokes it. *Laus vitae*, an 8,400-line poem, is an initiate's voyage through the human and pagan comedy; D'Annunzio rewrites the story of Paolo and Francesca in the play *Francesca da Rimini*; the very phrases used by D'Annunzio to categorize his works, "prose di romanzi" and "versi d'amore e di gloria," are taken from *Purgatorio* 26: "Versi d'amore e prose di romanzi / soverchiò tutti." The reference is to Dante's precursor Arnaut Daniel. For a discussion of *Francesca da Rimini* as

late to occupy such a position, and the charges of plagiarism in D'Annunzio's case seem to corroborate Bloom's notion of the impossibility of such "belated" ease. In fact, the critics disturbed by D'Annunzio's nonchalance take upon themselves the romantic anxiety of influence from which D'Annunzio himself seems not to suffer. Literary "inventions" are, for D'Annunzio, not private property but possibilities of language:

> Un verso perfetto è assoluto, immutabile, immortale; tiene in sé le parole con la coerenza d'un diamante; chiude il pensiero come in un cerchio preciso che nessuna forza mai riuscirà a rompere; diviene indipendente da ogni legame e da ogni dominio; non appartiene più all'artefice, ma è di tutti e di nessuno, come lo spazio, come la luce, come le cose immanenti e perpetue. Un pensiero esattamente espresso in un verso perfetto è un pensiero che già esisteva *preformato* nella oscura profondità della lingua.[5]

> [A perfect line of verse is absolute, immutable, immortal; it holds words within it with the coherence of a diamond; it encloses thought as though within a precise circle which no force will ever break; it becomes independent of all ties and all domination; it no longer belongs to the artifex but to everyone and no one, like space, like light, like all things immanent and perpetual. A thought precisely expressed in a perfect verse is a thought that already existed *preformed* in the obscure depths of language.]

Not in the depths of an individual psyche but in the depths of language—here lies D'Annunzio's modernity. Linguistic and literary materials and options circulate like space, like light, as though freed from the ties that anchored them to the past. Thus D'Annunzio is as free to combine the Renaissance patina of his

a critical response to Dante, see Paolo Valesio, "Dante e D'Annunzio," in *Quaderni Dannunziani* 3–4 (1988): 191–222.

5. Gabriele D'Annunzio, *Il piacere*, in *Prose di romanzi, Tutte le opere di Gabriele D'Annunzio*, ed. Egidio Bianchetti, 5th ed. (Milan: Mondadori, 1955), 1:150, hereafter cited in the text.

prose with a description of an airplane as he is to transpose a Maupassant tale into his native Pescara. Easy quotation becomes, rather than a sign of exhaustion or despair, an epigone's delight.

The scene of convalescence enacts the double movement of modernity whereby the past is canceled as diachrony in order that it may become the present: "The human figures that epitomize modernity," writes Paul de Man, "are defined by experiences such as childhood or convalescence, a freshness of perception that results from a slate wiped clear, from the absence of a past that has not yet had time to tarnish the immediacy of perception (although what is thus freshly discovered prefigures the end of this very freshness), of a past that, in the case of convalescence, is so threatening that it has to be forgotten."[6] The forgetfulness that characterizes the first moment in Baudelaire's, Nietzsche's, and D'Annunzio's portrayals of convalescence is followed by a second moment of total, and arbitrary, recall: "Comme il a été sur le point de tout oublier, il se souvient et veut avec ardeur se souvenir de tout" ["As he has been on the brink of total oblivion, he remembers, and fervently desires to remember, everything"].[7] So Baudelaire describes the convalescent in *Le peintre de la vie moderne.* D'Annunzio's Andrea Sperelli exhibits the same symptoms; at first a "creatura uscita da un fresco bagno letèo, immemore e vacua" ["creature emerged from a cool Lethean bath, empty and without memory"], the convalescent poet passes to a second moment of uncontrolled remembrance:

Ma questo periodo di visioni, di astrazioni, di intuizioni, di contemplazioni pure, questa specie di misticismo buddhistico e quasi direi cosmogonico, fu brevissimo. . . . Un giorno, nell'ora meridiana, mentre la vita delle cose pareva sospesa, il

6. Paul de Man, "Literary History and Literary Modernity," in *Blindness and Insight: Essays in the Rhetoric of Contemporary Criticism* (New York: Oxford University Press, 1971), 157. De Man discusses Baudelaire's *Peintre de la vie moderne* and Nietzsche's *Of the Use and Misuse of History for Life* and does not attribute delight to the writer who finds himself in the predicament of modernity.

7. Charles Baudelaire, *Le peintre de la vie moderne,* in *Oeuvres complètes,* ed. Claude Pichois, Bibliothèque de la Pléiade (Paris: Gallimard, 1976), 2:690; *The Painter of Modern Life and Other Essays,* trans. Jonathan Mayne (New York: Phaidon, 1964), 7, hereafter cited parenthetically in the text.

grande e terribile silenzio gli lasciò veder dentro, d'improvviso, abissi vertiginosi, bisogni inestinguibili, indistruttibili
ricordi, cumuli di sofferenza e di rimpianto, tutta la sua
miseria d'un tempo, tutti i vestigi del suo vizio, tutti gli
avanzi delle sue passioni. (*Il piacere,* 138–39)

[But this period of visions, of abstractions, of intuitions, of
pure contemplations, this sort of Buddhistic and I would
almost say cosmogonic mysticism was extremely brief. . . .
One day, at noon, while the life of things seemed suspended,
the great and terrible silence suddenly let him see inside
himself vertiginous abysses, inextinguishable needs, indestructible memories, accumulations of suffering and regret,
all of his misery of old, all the vestiges of his vice, and all the
leftovers of his passions.]

The tabula rasa of convalescence is covered with all the impressions
and vestiges of the past. The conflict between the two moments
would seem to defeat the aims of modernity. The new beginning,
the *tabula rasa* of the convalescent, figures modernity's break with
the past and, according to de Man, its rupture of genealogy.[8]
The child and the convalescent have nothing to remember. Yet
D'Annunzio's convalescent is also the last descendant of a noble
lineage (as are Giorgio Aurispa in *Trionfo della morte,* and the three
virgins of *Le vergini delle rocce*), "l'ultimo discendente d'una razza
intellettuale" ["the last descendant of an intellectual race"] (*Il
piacere,* 36). D'Annunzio's protagonists represent the culmination
of a genealogical line rather than its rupture. This predicament of
the protagonist mimes that of the decadent writer; as he attempts
to create a rupture he realizes that his "modernity" consists precisely
in the fact that he represents—he wishes to represent—the culmination of all that has gone before him. He is (and the theological
phrase is inevitable) both the beginning and the end. While in
philosophical terms, this predicament is an irresolvable paradox,
in the literary practice that results genealogy becomes a major

8. See de Man, "Literary History," 148. I am indebted to de Man's discussion
of modernity's desire to rupture genealogy in his seminar "The Aesthetic Theories
of Baudelaire and Diderot," Yale University, Spring 1983.

preoccupation, is thematized in order that it might be exorcized. The decadent rupture is caused by declaring oneself the end of the lineage, its culmination and fulfillment.

Decadent texts, then, encourage us to contemplate descriptions of genealogies, to admire a portrait gallery of aristocratic ancestors of both text and protagonist. Baudelaire occupies a position of honor in both Huysmans's and D'Annunzio's galleries, flanked by Verlaine, Flaubert, and in D'Annunzio's case, the English romantics and Wagner. Baudelaire's texts are recycled, reread by both Huysmans and D'Annunzio: *A rebours* has been read, at the text's own suggestion, as an enactment of the prose poem "Any where out of the world," and Baudelaire is cited lovingly as Des Esseintes's favorite author.[9] D'Annunzio makes his debt explicit in *L'Innocente,* citing the canonical words "dovunque fuori del mondo!" ["anywhere out of the world!"], and Baudelaire's presence is even stronger in *Il poema paradisiaco* and *Il piacere.*[10] Baudelaire thus seems to stand serenely as the legitimate and legitimating father of decadentism. Yet as we gaze (and we are still following the pebble path strewn by the text), this portrait begins to assume the demented and demonic shapes of Lombroso's genealogical trees, in which the horror of origins disfigures even the most illustrious lineage.[11]

9. "Son admiration pour cet écrivain était sans borne. . . . Et plus Des Esseintes relisait Baudelaire, plus il reconnaissait un indicible charme à cet écrivain qui, dans un temps où le vers ne servait plus qu'à peindre l'aspect extérieur des êtres et des choses, était parvenu à exprimer l'inexprimable, grâce à une langue musculeuse et charnue, qui plus que tout autre, possédait cette merveilleuse puissance de fixer, avec une étrange santé d'expressions, les états morbides les plus fuyants, les plus tremblés, des esprits epuisés et des âmes tristes." ["His admiration for this writer knew no bounds. . . . The more Des Esseintes re-read his Baudelaire, the more he appreciated the indescribable charm of this writer who, at a time when verse no longer served any purpose except to depict the external appearance of creatures and things, had succeeded in expressing the inexpressible—thanks to a solid, sinewy style which, more than any other, possessed that remarkable quality, the power to define in curiously healthy terms the most fugitive and ephemeral of the unhealthy conditions of weary spirits and melancholy souls."] J. K. Huysmans, *A rebours*, ed. Marc Fumaroli (1882; Paris: Gallimard, 1977), 260–62; *Against Nature*, trans. Robert Baldick (1959; rpt. Middlesex, Eng.: Penguin, 1979), 146–48.

10. Gabriele D'Annunzio, *L'Innocente*, in *Prose di romanzi*, 1:417.

11. Lombroso's studies are literal illustrations of *pudenda origo*; see *L'uomo di genio in rapporto alla psichiatria, alla storia, ed all'estetica*, 6th ed. (Turin: Fratelli

Harold Bloom's serious play on influence as a sort of influenza assumes literal form, for "Baudelaire" enters into the semiosis of decadence as both the texts that bear his signature and Baudelaire himself as text.[12] Baudelaire becomes a sign when his fatal illness is mythified as the most horrifying of all writers' fates. In this double portrait we find both a reassuring likeness—Baudelaire's texts as legitimate father—and a disquieting otherness—Baudelaire as text, as paralysis and aphasia.

We have, however, not yet abandoned Hansel and Gretel in the woods, nor have we led them happily home. The problem posed by the fable, in fact, is not only how to return to the father but how to kill the mother. In the fairy tale there are two paths, a first marked with pebbles visible in the moonlight and a second laid with bread crumbs. This second path is consumed and erased, and the siblings (and, I suggest, the text) end up in the clutches of the witch, the bad mother in disguise. Our analogy ends before the happy ending in which the witch is killed, and as the children discover upon their return, their displaced desire to kill the mother has hit home—the stepmother is dead as well. By reading the texts of Baudelaire, Huysmans, D'Annunzio, and Nietzsche as readings

Bocca, 1894). Lombroso includes in an appendix the genealogical tree of the Roman Caesars and that of the Spanish dynasty from 1357 to 1700. We may take the latter tree as an example: the dynasty stems from Pedro I of Portugal, "proavo lunatico, crudele" ["lunatic, cruel ancestor"], who belongs to the category of "criminali pazzi morali" ["morally mad criminals"] and produces Isabella di Portogallo, "che fu pazza negli ultimi anni" ["who was mad in her last years"]; Maria Tudor, "pazza isterica sterile" ["sterile, hysterical madwoman"]; Carlo V, "geniale, melanconico, epilettico . . . mangiatore e bevitore con denti brutti" ["genial, melancholic, epileptic, a great eater and drinker with bad teeth"], who belongs to the categories of "pazzi ed imbecilli" ["madmen and imbeciles"], "epilettici" ["epileptics"] and "geniali" ["the genial"]. The dynasty ends with Carlo II, "ultimo della dinastia, a 10 anni non si reggeva in piedi, melanconico, sposò una francese senza prole, una tedesca senza prole, a 35 anni perdè i capelli e i cigli, era epilettico e morì nel 1700" ["the last of the dynasty, at the age of ten he could not stand up, was melancholic, married a childless Frenchwoman, a childless German, at the age of thirty-five lost his hair and eyelashes, was epileptic and died in 1700"] (L'uomo di genio, table xviii). We are not so far from Giorgio Aurispa's description of his family.

12. "The Cartesian reductions of time and space brought upon us the further blight of the negative aspect of poetic influence, of influenza in the realm of literature, as the influx of an epidemic of anxiety." Bloom, 38.

of one another, thus by following the fatherly path, we may perceive traces of the other, effaced path whose erasure led to a mother: a ritual expulsion of woman is followed by her return in grotesque form. That return may call into question the genealogical rhetoric that employs the language of fatherhood, for the scene of her return is also the scene of artistic and philosophic creation: convalescence.[13]

The scene of convalescence to which this text will repeatedly return is that of Andrea Sperelli. In the second book of *Il piacere,* Sperelli retreats to a *locus amoenus,* Schifanoia, to convalesce after a duel in which he had, we are told, received a "mortale ferita" ["mortal wound"]. The convalescent is reborn—"la convalescenza è una purificazione e un rinascimento" ["convalescence is a purification and a rebirth"]—and discovers poetry and his own poetic vocation. This rediscovered vocation would seem to replace Sperelli's vocation in book 1 as a womanizing dandy:

L'Arte! L'Arte!—Ecco l'Amante fedele, sempre giovine, immortale. . . . Come le sue mani avevan potuto oziare e lascivire su i corpi delle femmine dopo aver sentito erompere dalle dita una forma sostanziale? Come, infine, i suoi sensi avean potuto indebolirsi e pervertirsi nella bassa lussuria dopo essere stati illuminati da una sensibilità che coglieva nelle apparenze le linee invisibili, percepiva l'impercettibile, indovinava i pensieri nascosti della Natura? (*Il piacere,* 146–47)

[Art! Art!—She is the faithful Lover, forever young, immortal. . . . How could his hands have lain idle and lascivious on the bodies of females after having felt substantial form erupt from his fingers? How, finally, could his senses have weakened and perverted themselves in base lasciviousness after having been illuminated by a sensitivity that grasped invisible lines in appearances, that perceived the imperceptible, that divined the hidden thoughts of Nature?]

13. It is striking that, according to the *OED,* the verb *to convalesce* did not appear in English dictionaries or in ordinary English usage until the nineteenth century.

The lapsed aesthete returns to his true faith. Like Saint Augustine, Sperelli leaves behind him his *nugae* in order to devote himself to a "purer" contemplation: convalescence is a sort of secular conversion. As Kenneth Burke has noted in his reading of Augustine, the rhetoric of conversion inevitably evokes its dialectical counterpart—perversion.[14] Sperelli's dallyings are thus a prerequisite to his conversion to art. Yet Sperelli's devoted gaze soon drifts from art, the faithful lover, to Maria Ferres, *turris eburnea:* the expelled woman returns in the sacralized guise of a mother Mary. Dedication of poems to her similarly drifts toward an abdication of poetic voice as the narrative shifts from the third person to the "I" of Maria Ferres's diary.

This brief and already interpretive summary allows us to raise several questions: What is the relation between convalescence and creation? Why is woman expelled from the scene of convalescence, and more interesting, why and how does she return? And finally, where does convalescence take place? Responses to these questions will be drawn from descriptions of convalescence in the texts of Baudelaire, Huysmans, D'Annunzio, and Nietzsche, which will be unraveled so as to construct a text of which those descriptions are fragments. Convalescence as the scene of artistic and philosophical creation is an ideologeme of decadent texts, a narrative that lies between texts.

The Liquidation of the Crowd

Convalescence itself is a space in-between, a hazy yet paradoxically crystal-clear state between sickness and health. Introduced as a third term in the rhetoric of sickness and health, convalescence becomes the vehicle for a series of in-between states. Physiologically ambiguous—not sick-unto-death yet not quite healthy either—the convalescent is also socially ambiguous. Typically, he is a

14. See Kenneth Burke, *The Rhetoric of Religion: Studies in Logology* (1961; rpt. Berkeley: University of California Press, 1970), as well as his article on Djuna Barnes, "Version, Con-, Per-, and In-: Thoughts on Djuna Barnes' Novel *Nightwood*," in *Language as Symbolic Action* (Berkeley: University of California Press, 1966), 240–53.

member of a historically dislocated aristocracy, a marginal and waning class, which is itself a third term between bourgeoisie and proletariat. In the texts of Huysmans and D'Annunzio the aristocrat's historical dislocation is mimed by the convalescent's topographical dislocation: both Andrea Sperelli and Jean Des Esseintes flee the city, suffering from a "dégoût du réel" which is also a "dégoût du social." Yet in Baudelaire's 1863 essay, *Le peintre de la vie moderne*, the convalescent's domain appears to be the social world represented synecdochically by that great nineteenth-century obsession, the urban crowd. D'Annunzio, who did not shy away from the urban crowd either in his art (notably, in *Il fuoco*) or in his life (in particular, in his dialogues with the crowd at Fiume) excludes the crowd from his description of convalescence, a description that in all other respects employs a "Baudelairean" rhetoric. We may uncover some reasons for this exclusion by placing the Baudelairean text in dialogue with *Il piacere*.

As we have seen, the convalescent is a figure for the poet in *Il piacere;* in *Le peintre de la vie moderne* it is a painter who is convalescent: "Supposez un artiste qui serait toujours, spirituellement, à l'état du convalescent, et vous aurez la clef du caractère de M. G." (*Le peintre,* 690) ["Imagine an artist who was always, spiritually, in the condition of that convalescent, and you will have the key to the nature of Monsieur G." (Mayne, 7)]. M. Constantin Guys assumes many masks—artist, man of the world, child—but the couple that interests us here is "l'homme des foules—convalescent." Baudelaire has, of course, been reading Edgar Allan Poe, whose story "The Man of the Crowd" serves as a model for his description of Guys. I quote Baudelaire's account in full, since we will have occasion to return to it:

Vous souvenez-vous d'un tableau (en vérité, c'est un tableau!) écrit par la plus puissante plume de cette époque, et qui a pour titre *L'Homme des foules?* Derrière la vitre d'un café, un convalescent, contemplant la foule avec jouissance, se mêle par la pensée, à toutes les pensées qui s'agitent autour de lui. Revenu récemment des ombres de la mort, il aspire avec délices tous les germes et tous les effluves de la vie; comme il a été sur le point de tout oublier, il se souvient et veut avec ardeur se souvenir de tout. Finalement, il se précipite à travers cette foule à la recherche d'un inconnu dont la physiognomie entrevue l'a, en un clin d'oeil, fasciné. La curiosité est devenue une passion fatale, irrésistible! (*Le peintre*, 689–90)

[Do you remember a picture (it really is a picture!), painted— or rather written—by the most powerful pen of our age, and entitled *The Man of the Crowd?* In the window of a coffee-house there sits a convalescent, pleasurably absorbed in gazing at the crowd, and mingling, through the medium of thought, in the turmoil of thought that surrounds him. But lately returned from the valley of the shadow of death, he is rapturously breathing in all the odours and essences of life; as he has been on the brink of total oblivion, he remembers, and fervently desires to remember, everything. Finally he hurls himself headlong into the midst of the throng, in pursuit of an unknown, half-glimpsed countenance that has, on an instant, bewitched him. Curiosity has become a fatal, irresistible passion! (Mayne, 7)]

In coupling convalescent and "l'homme des foules" under the umbrella term "Constantin Guys," Baudelaire has already interpreted Poe, for Poe's man of the crowd is not the convalescent who observes the crowd but the man pursued and observed *by* the convalescent, "the type and genius of true crime."[15] Baudelaire's reassignment of roles so that the convalescent himself is the man of the crowd can be read as an identification of the artist with pathology. "Baudelaire," remarked Walter Benjamin in his brilliant essay on the flaneur, "wrote no detective story because, given the structure of his instincts, it was impossible for him to identify with the detective."[16] Indeed, even in his reading he obliterates the detective's role, truncating his account of Poe at the point when the convalescent merges into the crowd. He continues with a writing of the man of the crowd's relationship *to* the crowd which differs greatly from Poe's story.

15. Edgar Allan Poe, "The Man of the Crowd," in *Great Short Works of Edgar Allan Poe*, ed. G. R. Thompson (New York: Harper & Row, 1970), 272.
16. Walter Benjamin, *Charles Baudelaire: A Lyric Poet in the Era of High Capitalism*, trans. Harry Zohn (London: New Left Books, 1973), 43.

Like Andrea Sperelli, who moves to a paradisiacal garden on the margins of society, Constantin Guys occupies a liminal position within the crowd. Guys's goal and pleasure is to "voir le monde, être au centre du monde et rester caché au monde" (*Le peintre*, 692) ["to see the world, to be at the centre of the world, and yet to remain hidden from the world" (Mayne, 9)]. The three activities— to see, to be at the center, and yet not to be seen—are simultaneous rather than sequential, and yet the third term arises suddenly, paradoxically, from the previous two desires, creating a third space, which absorbs them. Thus M. Guys is not an outside observer who views the crowd from a distance, nor does he participate wholly in it. Instead, he is an outside observer inside the social sphere. "L'observateur," writes Baudelaire, "est un *prince* qui jouit partout de son incognito" (*Le peintre, 692*) ["The spectator is a *prince* who everywhere rejoices in his incognito" (Mayne, 9)]. This third space, inside yet outside, is occupied by a sort of secret agent; yet unlike the prince evoked by Baudelaire, he is an agent with allegiances to neither term—neither the crowd through which he wanders nor the institutions that control the crowd's meanderings. [17] His only confidant is his art. The convalescent assumes as many perspectives as he does masks, artfully dodging definition and aspiring to a stance that would be both inside and outside of his class and its ideology.

Yet like the secret agent's, the convalescent's position is precarious. Not healthy enough to participate in the social mechanism (in particular, to work), yet not sick enough to be institutionalized, the convalescent teeters between two modes of falling back into social organization. It is this that he shares with the dandy of the same essay and with the wine drinker and hashish eater of *Les*

---

17. The crowd, of course, was an area of special interest to nineteenth-century writers and criminologists. Benjamin links the appearance of pocket-sized volumes called physiologies to this aspect of urban life and quotes a turn-of-the-century police report: "'It is almost impossible,' wrote a Parisian secret agent in 1798, 'to maintain good behaviour in a thickly populated area when an individual is, so to speak, unknown to all others and thus does not have to blush in front of anyone.' Here the masses appear as the asylum that shields an asocial person from his persecutors. Of all the menacing aspects of the masses, this one became apparent first. It is at the origin of the detective story" (Benjamin, 40).

paradis artificiels. These "hommes déclassés, dégoûtés, désoeuvrés" ["idle, disgusted, and déclassé men"] all belong to a special ward of "les malades" and are similarly on leave from the demands and restrictions laid upon the healthy citizen:

> Or, nous connaissons assez la nature humaine pour savoir qu'un homme qui peut, avec une cuillerée de confiture, se procurer instantanément tous les biens du ciel et de la terre, n'en gagnera jamais la millième partie par le travail. Se figure-t-on un État dont les citoyens s'enivreraient de hachisch? Quels citoyens! quels guerriers! quels législateurs!

> [We understand enough of human nature to know that a man who, with a spoonful of conserve, can instantaneously procure for himself all the benefits of heaven and earth, will never earn a thousandth part of these by toil. Can one imagine a State of which all the citizens intoxicated themselves with hashish? What citizens, what warriors and legislators!][18]

The effects of hashish, it is true, are presented as ultimately pernicious and debilitating. The hashish eater's artificial convalescence edges toward a relapse not so much because hashish prevents one from becoming a good citizen but because it annihilates the will to create and to produce: "A quoi bon, en effet, travailler, labourer, écrire, fabriquer quoi que ce soit, quand on peut emporter le paradis d'un seul coup?" ["Indeed, what is the point of working, laboring, writing, making anything at all when one can obtain paradise in a single stroke?"].[19] The work that is valued is not the labor of the common man—for him even wine is reserved for Sundays and forgetfulness—but the work of artistic creation, a work of which the wine drinker is superbly capable. "Le vin" opens with the song wine sings to the working man but closes with a parable of a guitarist who, intoxicated, intoxicates his audience with his master-

18. Charles Baudelaire, "Le poème du hachisch," *Les paradis artificiels,* in *Oeuvres complètes,* 1:438; *The Poem of Hashish,* in *The Essence of Laughter and Other Essays, Journals, and Letters,* ed. Peter Quennell, trans. Norman Cameron (New York: Meridian Books, 1956), 102.

19. Baudelaire, "Du vin et du hachisch," in *Les paradis artificiels,* 397.

ful playing. Both intoxicants, wine and hashish, provide the necessary stimulus, "le développement poétique excessif de l'homme"
["the excessive poetic development of man"],[20] but wine does not
impair the will and desire to represent. The wine drinker, hashish
eater, and convalescent exchange symptomatologies: intoxication
is one of the symptoms of convalescence, the intoxicated partake
of the convalescent's creative urge, and all three experience thought
as an invasion. Similar analogies are engendered by similar discourses; the disguised prince of *Le peintre de la vie moderne* becomes
in "Du vin et du hachisch" the Holy Ghost. Wine creates, in a
typically decadent play on its theological value, "pour ainsi dire,
une troisième personne, opération mystique, où l'homme naturel
et le vin, le dieu animal et le dieu végetal, jouent le rôle du Père
et du Fils dans la Trinité; ils engendrent un Saint-Esprit, qui est
l'homme supérieur, lequel procède également des deux"[21] ["a third
person, as it were, a mystical operation in which the natural man
and wine, the animal god and the vegetal god, play the role of
Father and Son in the Trinity. They engender a Holy Spirit who
is the superior man who derives equally from the two of them"].
Once again a third term is introduced which encompasses and
surpasses the two terms upon which it depends. M. Guys's three
goals could, in fact, be said to be a secularization of this triad, if
to see the world is the Father's prerogative, to be at its center the
Son's, and to be mysteriously hidden from the world is the Holy
Ghost's privilege.

We have assumed, following and falling prey to the suggestion
of the text, that the world in which the convalescent sees yet is not
seen is the social world evoked by *la foule,* an urban crowd. Yet
this crowd turns out to be not a collection of human faces and
forms but a sort of crowd effect, the watery motion of "le fleuve de
la vitalité" ["the river of vitality"]:

> La foule est son domaine, comme l'air est celui de l'oiseau,
> comme l'eau celui du poisson. Sa passion et sa profession, c'est
> *d'épouser la foule.* Pour le parfait flâneur, pour l'observateur
> passionné, c'est une immense jouissance que d'élire domicile

20. Ibid.
21. Ibid., 387.

dans le nombre, dans l'ondoyant, dans le mouvement, dans le fugitif et l'infini. (*Le peintre,* 691)

[The crowd is his element, as the air is that of birds and water of fishes. His passion and his profession are to become one flesh with the crowd. For the perfect *flâneur,* for the passionate spectator, it is an immense joy to set up house in the heart of the multitude, amid the ebb and flow of movement, in the midst of the fugitive and the infinite. (Mayne, 9)]

Benjamin's remark that, for Victor Hugo, "the crowd really is a spectacle of nature" would seem to apply to Baudelaire's description as well, for the convalescent takes up his abode in a watery realm of abstractions.[22] Undulating, horizonless movement associates the crowd with the sea; the grammatical femininity of *la foule* is foregrounded, awakened by the association of water and archetypal femininity. This association is reinforced by Guys's professional passion to marry the crowd, the *jouissance* that follows his marriage, as well as by "la démarche des femmes onduleuses" ["the undulous gait of the women"], which appears in the subsequent paragraph when shadowy forms begin to surface from the crowd. Contact between convalescent and crowd is erotic:[23]

L'amateur de la vie fait du monde sa famille, comme l'amateur du beau sexe compose sa famille de toutes les beautés trouvées, trouvables et introuvables; comme l'amateur de tableaux vit dans une société enchantée de rêves peints sur toile. Ainsi l'amoureux de la vie universelle entre dans la foule comme dans un immense réservoir d'électricité. (*Le peintre,* 692)

[The lover of life makes the whole world his family, just like the lover of the fair sex who builds up his family from all the beautiful women that he has ever found, or that are—or are

22. Benjamin, 62.
23. Benjamin notes that Baudelaire's sonnet "A une passante" "presents the crowd not as the refuge of a criminal but as that of love which eludes the poet. One may say that it deals with the function of the crowd not in the life of the citizen but in the life of the erotic person" (45).

not—to be found; or the lover of pictures who lives in a
magical society of dreams painted on canvas. Thus the lover
of universal life enters into the crowd as though it were an
immense reservoir of electrical energy. (Mayne, 9)]

The convalescent's relation to a presumably human multitude is
the least human of these analogies; rather than composing a family
or an "enchanted society," he merges into an undifferentiated
vastness. This merging is not, however, a loss of self for in the
same moment he becomes a mirror of the crowd, a "kaleidoscope
doué de conscience" ["kaleidoscope gifted with consciousness"] able
to represent multiplicity to his own consciousness, to absorb and
become the vastness observed. The convalescent's consciousness is
the only consciousness present: "C'est un *moi* insatiable du *non-moi*"
(*Le peintre*, 692) ["He is an 'I' with an insatiable appetite for the
non 'I'" (Mayne, 9)]. By ingesting the *non-moi*, the convalescent
multiplies himself (just as the hashish eater becomes multiple by
ingesting hashish), and the multiplication is enacted by the text
itself. Names for Constantin Guys proliferate: "l'artiste," "l'homme
du monde," "l'homme des foules," "l'enfant," "le convalescent,"
"le génie," "le dandy," "l'amoureux," "le prince," and "le peintre
de la vie moderne." The undifferentiated crowd is filtered through
Constantin Guys's consciousness to become a crowd of names.

Andrea Sperelli, a man of the world, lover, dandy, a count if not
a prince, enters a convalescence that is also "puerizia" ["infancy"],
"adolescenza" ["adolescence"], and the awakening of genius. Like
Baudelaire's convalescent, he is subject to congestion and fevers; he,
too, is in search of modernity. The only term to have disappeared is
"l'homme des foules," for there is no mention of an urban crowd
in this convalescent's domain. One might, as Mario Ricciardi does,
interpret the exclusion as an evasive and ultimately reactionary
move, a polemical gesture that sweeps away the progressive causes
that crowds so often represented in the nineteenth century.[24] To

24. Mario Ricciardi, *Coscienza e struttura nella prosa di D'Annunzio* (Turin:
Giappichelli, 1970). Ricciardi identifies the displacement of the urban crowd
to the countryside as a polemical move that aims to oppose (ahistorical) peasant
masses to the (historical) appearance of the proletarian urban crowd. D'Annunzio's refusal to accept the existence of the urban proletariat would thus be
motivated by a refusal to accept its political goals. The peasant masses are,

be sure, the crowd is a politically charged topic; a literary description of it in the nineteenth century, especially after 1848 and the Paris Commune, cannot be neutral. To espouse the crowd meant to espouse a cause, much as, to give a contemporary example, a lyrical description of a nuclear reactor would be interpreted as a political move. Indeed, the convalescent's espousal of the crowd in *Le peintre de la vie moderne* can be read as a sign of Baudelaire's radical, utopian impulse. The undifferentiated vastness of the crowd implies a kind of equality among elements, an equality that cannot fail to evoke political equality as well. In that same essay, the political valence comes to the fore in a strikingly nonpolitical context:

> Un artiste ayant le sentiment parfait de la forme, mais accoutumé à exercer surtout sa mémoire et son imagination, se trouve alors comme assailli par une émeute de details, qui tous demandent justice avec la furie d'une foule amoureuse d'égalité absolue. (*Le peintre*, 698–99)

> [An artist with a perfect sense of form but one accustomed to relying above all on his memory and his imagination will find himself at the mercy of a riot of details all clamouring for

Ricciardi writes, "exalted as the genuine and immutable expression of the pure values of the race and of the nation. Thus D'Annunzio prepares the myth of the juxtaposition between the pure and natural peasant world and the corrupt and artificial world of the industrial city" (83). While I agree that this displacement of the urban crowd is a polemical gesture, I would add that the polemic might also be directed toward the "dati del reale" that preoccupy Ricciardi. The representation of masses of peasants rather than workers might be interpreted as a reading of Italian political reality in the late nineteenth century, a reality which did *not* correspond to that of the more advanced industrial societies of France and England. D'Annunzio's representations of peasants emphasize the specificity and, in relation to the French and English models, the backwardness of Italy. The myth of "the pure and natural peasant world," opposed to the corrupt industrial city, is Ricciardi's rather than D'Annunzio's. The "pure and natural" peasant world is presented by D'Annunzio (in *Terra vergine, Le novelle della Pescara, Trionfo della morte*) as sickness and degeneration. D'Annunzio is interested in civilization and artificiality, not in bemoaning a lost preindustrial purity.

justice with the fury of a mob in love with absolute equality. (Mayne, 16)]

A riot of details turns into an angry crowd that demands justice and equality; a formal problem becomes a political one. This "intrusion" of the political onto the scene of the artist's activity stands as an emblem not only of the artist in general but of the nineteenth-century writer faced with the literarization of the crowd. As a counterexample to Baudelaire, we might cite Manzoni, whose *I promessi sposi* is marked, in Gramsci's words, by a "paternalismo padreternale." The crowd is a gauge of political temperament; in his novel Manzoni represented the urban crowd as a plague-ridden mob. In life, Manzoni was an agoraphobic; crowds brought on epileptoid seizures, one of which he took to be a sign from God that he should convert to Catholicism. The text of his life can be interpreted through his literary texts, for they are grounded in the same ideological matrix.[25] D'Annunzio's case is more complex, for as we have said, the crowd appears in several guises in his novels and life. Its exclusion from *Il piacere* cannot be read simply as the incompatibility of the crowd with the scene of artistic creation, for the artist's relationship to the crowd is an important theme of *Il fuoco* and of his speeches at Fiume. Nor, it seems to me, can a developmental scheme be evoked, not because I agree with Croce's denial that development ever took place but because such chronological explanations, as we have learned from Nietzsche, often mask disturbing contradictions. The reasons for the crowd's exclusion begin to appear when we read D'Annunzio through Baudelaire and when we place D'Annunzio's other novels in dialogue with *Il piacere*.

It is possible to perceive the ghost of a human multitude in the description of Sperelli's convalescence, a multitude whose humanity has, however, been liquidated:

25. Manzoni's case did not go unexplored by Lombrosians. In 1898 Paolo Bellezza wrote a case study, *Genio e follia di Alessandro Manzoni*. To my knowledge, more recent psychoanalytic studies of Manzoni have not dealt with this nexus between his art and life. The existing studies focus on the Monaca di Monza. See Michel David's chapter on Manzoni in *Letteratura e psicanalisi* (Milan: Mursia, 1967), 140–44 and 317–60, and Ferruccio Ulivi's chapter "Manzoni e la psicanalisi," in *Manzoni: Storia e provvidenza* (Rome: Bonacci, 1974).

Parevagli d'essere entrato in una forma più elementare. Il passato per la sua memoria aveva una sola lontananza, come per la vista il cielo stellato è un campo uguale e diffuso sebbene gli astri sien diversamente distanti. I tumulti si pacificavano, il fango scendeva all'imo, l'anima facevasi monda; ed egli rientrava nel grembo della natura madre, sentivasi da lei maternamente infondere la bontà e la forza.

Ospitato da sua cugina nella villa di Schifanoia, Andrea Sperelli si riaffacciava all'esistenza in conspetto del mare. (*Il piacere,* 135–36)

[It seemed to him that he had entered a more elementary form. The past had a single distance for his memory, just as for sight the starry skies are an equal and diffuse field even though the stars are at different distances. The tumults calmed, the mud sank to the bottom, his soul was cleansed. And he reentered the womb of mother nature and felt himself maternally infused by her with goodness and strength.

The guest of his cousin in the villa at Schifanoia, Andrea Sperelli returned to existence again in sight of the sea.]

Baudelaire's convalescent sat behind the window of a cafe with the crowd before him; Sperelli faces a different vastness, the sea. Within the context of a description that closely follows the Baudelairean rhetoric of convalescence, the substitution of sea for crowd is an interpretation of Baudelaire's text. The crowd does indeed become a spectacle of nature. Moreover, it seems that the feminine valence of Baudelaire's crowd has been retained, through a paronomastic play on *madre*/*mare* (the paronomasia is, of course, even stronger in the French *mer*/*mère*). D'Annunzio expels the social element by following the language used to describe the crowd's effect, thereby emptying the crowd of any potentially social quality. Only kaleidoscopic consciousness remains:

Il mare aveva sempre per lui una parola profonda, piena di rivelazioni subitanee, d'illuminazioni improvvise, di significazioni inaspettate. Gli scopriva nella segreta anima un'ulcera ancor viva sebben nascosta e glie la faceva sanguinare; ma il balsamo poi era più soave. Gli scoteva nel cuore una chimera dormente e glie la incitava così ch'ei ne sentisse di nuovo le unghie e il rostro; ma glie la uccideva poi e glie la seppelliva nel cuore per sempre. Gli svegliava nella memoria una ricordanza e glie l'avvivava così ch'ei sofferisse tutta l'amarezza del rimpianto verso le cose irrimediabilmente fuggite; ma gli prodigava poi la dolcezza d'un oblìo senza fine. Nulla entro quell'anima rimaneva celato, al conspetto del gran consolatore. Alla guisa che una forte corrente elettrica rende luminosi i metalli e rivela la loro essenza dal color della loro fiamma, la virtù del mare illuminava e rivelava tutte le potenze e le potenzialità di quell'anima umana. (*Il piacere,* 140)

[The sea had always held a profound word for him, full of sudden revelations, unexpected illuminations, unprecedented meanings. The sea revealed to him an ulcer in his secret soul, an ulcer still alive even though hidden, and made it bleed. But the balm was gentle later. The sea reawakened a sleeping chimera in his heart and incited it so that he once again felt its claws and beak. But later the sea killed it and buried it in his heart forever. The sea awoke a recollection in his memory and revived it so that he suffered all the bitterness of regret toward things irremediably gone. But later it bestowed upon him the sweetness of an endless forgetfulness. Nothing remained concealed within that soul as it faced the great consoler. Just as a strong electrical current makes metals luminous and reveals their essence by the color of their flame, so did the virtue of the sea illuminate and reveal all the powers and potentialities of that human soul.]

D'Annunzio's sea, like Baudelaire's crowd, is a reservoir of electricity that acts upon and illuminates the subject who will record these jolts as poems or sketches. This electrical current passes from Poe through Baudelaire to D'Annunzio, welding together their descriptions of convalescence.[26] But Baudelaire acts as a conductor

26. In Poe's story, we read: "For some months I had been ill in health, but was now convalescent, and, with returning strength, found myself in one of those happy moods which are so precisely the converse of *ennui*—moods of the keenest appetency, when the film from the mental vision departs—the αχλυς ος πριν επηεν—and the intellect, electrified, surpasses as greatly its everyday

in yet another sense, for the "continuous tides of population" and the "tumultuous sea of human heads" which appear in "The Man of the Crowd" have, through Baudelaire's mediation, become simply tides and sea.[27] The crowd is banished from the D'Annunzian scene of convalescence in order to place an electrified intellect at center stage. The fevers and congestion that afflict the convalescent and sharpen his consciousness turn sight into vision. The crowd is still necessary in Baudelaire's text as the object of that vision, as the locus of the *non-moi*. D'Annunzio goes one step further: he internalizes that pathology so that observer and observed are truly one; it is the multiplicity of the self, the *non-moi* within the *moi*, which

condition as does the vivid yet candid reason of Leibnitz, the mad and flimsy rhetoric of Gorgias" (262). The image of an electric current is suppressed in the 1894 version of *Il piacere*, which D'Annunzio prepared for Georges Hérelle's 1894 French translation. It is striking that almost all the passages I have cited as evidence of a genealogical connection are deleted from this edition of *Il piacere*, among them, the entire opening paragraph of book 2, beginning "La convalescenza è una purificazione e un rinascimento" and ending "le ali alle chimere della fantasia" (135); the passage beginning "Il desiderio aveva abbandonato il suo regno" until "la causa del non mai provato godimento" (137); the sentence beginning "Alla guisa che una forte corrente elettrica" (140); the entire passage beginning "L'ideale avvelena ogni possesso imperfetto" until "Meglio morire!" (145–48). This last deletion thereby excludes Sperelli's sonnet, his exclamations concerning what I have called his conversion to "l'Arte . . . l'Amante fedele," as well as his fears that his intelligence may not have remained intact following his illness. (This passage will be discussed in relation to Baudelairean *influenza* in chapter 3.) Also excluded are his disquisition on aesthetics (149–51); the passage in which Giulia Moceto and her lack of "la douce barbe feminine" are discussed (244–47); and the misogynist dinner episode (254–57). The last two exclusions could be explained as moralistic ones; in fact, in a letter to Hérelle, cited by Ivanos Ciani, D'Annunzio assured his friend and translator that he had suppressed the most scandalous passages. Yet the other passages I have cited cannot be considered scandalous from the point of view of sexual mores. It is tempting to speculate that D'Annunzio may have felt his "French connections" were too evident in the excluded passages. The problem with such an interpretation is, of course, that D'Annunzio was not wont to show any anxiety whatsoever with regard to possible accusations of plagiarism. For the 1894 version of *Il piacere*, see *Il piacere nella stesura preparata dall'autore per l'edizione francese del 1894*, ed. Ivanos Ciani (Milan: Mondadori, 1976). Georgina Harding's translation of *Il piacere*, *The Child of Pleasure*, is in fact a translation of the 1894 Italian version, rather than of the original Italian.

27. Poe, 262.

is observed. While Baudelaire's convalescent is "un miroir aussi immense que cette foule" ["a mirror as immense as this crowd"], D'Annunzio's convalescent sees himself mirrored in the immensity of the sea. Andrea Sperelli's convalescence thus prepares the ground for a later D'Annunzian convalescent, Tullio Hermil, "il multanime" ["many-souled"] of *L'Innocente*.

But there is yet another reason for the liquidation of the crowd in this novel about erotic pleasure, a motivation that we can reconstruct only through recourse to other D'Annunzian texts. The crowd reappears in D'Annunzio's novels like a hysterical symptom moving from one part of the body politic to another. Expelled from the description of convalescence in *Il piacere,* the urban crowd returns in *Il fuoco* and, more interestingly for the present discussion, in the third and last book of the *Romanzi della Rosa, Trionfo della morte.* In *Trionfo della morte,* the urban crowd returns in displaced form as an archaic mob of peasants who descend in droves upon the sanctuary at Casalbordino. Identified more frequently by the pejorative term *torma* than by the neutral label *folla,* it is metonymically linked to that other element excluded from the scene of convalescence, woman, or rather, a particular part of woman. Baudelaire's crowd and D'Annunzio's sea are, as we have noted, characterized as "feminine" elements, as comforting, even motherly, movement. The peasant mob of *Trionfo della morte* might also be said to have a feminine valence, though of a different sort, for it appears as a sign of the woman's illness, a synecdoche of Ippolita. The description of this horde is a congeries of human vice and deformation:

> Era uno spettacolo meraviglioso e terribile, inopinato, dissimile ad ogni aggregazione già veduta di cose e di genti, composto di mescolanze così strane aspre e diverse che superava i più torbidi sogni prodotti dall'incubo. Tutte le brutture dell'ilota eterno, tutti i vizii turpi, tutti gli stupori; tutti gli spasimi e le deformazioni della carne battezzata, tutte le lacrime del pentimento, tutte le risa della crapula; la follia, la cupidigia, l'astuzia, la lussuria, la frode, l'ebetudine, la paura, la stanchezza mortale, l'indifferenza impietrita, la disperazione taciturna; i cori sacri, gli ululi degli ossessi, i berci dei funamboli, i rintocchi della campane, gli squilli delle

trombe, i ragli, i muggiti, i nitriti; i fuochi crepitanti sotto
le caldaie, i cumuli dei frutti e dei dolciumi, le mostre degli
utensili, dei tessuti, delle armi, dei gioielli, dei rosarii; le
danze oscene delle saltatrici, le convulsioni degli epilettici, le
percosse dei rissanti, le fughe dei ladri inseguiti a traverso la
calca, la suprema schiuma delle corruttele portata fuori dai
vicoli immondi delle città remote e rovesciata su una molti-
tudine ignara e attonita; come tafani sul bestiame, nuvoli
di parassiti implacabili su una massa compatta incapace di
difendersi; tutte le basse tentazioni agli appetiti brutali, tutti
gli inganni alla semplicità e alla stupidezza, tutte le ciurmerie
e le impudicizie professate in pieno meriggio; tutte le mesco-
lanze erano là, ribollivano, fermentavano, intorno alla Casa
della Vergine.[28]

[It was a marvelous and terrible spectacle, unheard of, unlike
any conglomeration ever seen before, whether of men or
things; a spectacle composed of mixtures so strange, so harsh
and incongruous, that it exceeded the most troubled dreams
produced by an incubus. All the ugliness of the eternal Helot,
all the foul vices, all the stupors; all the spasms and all the
deformities of baptized flesh, all the tears of repentance, all the
mockery of gluttony; insanity, cupidity, cunning, lewdness,
fraud, stupidity, fear, mortal fatigue, stony indifference, silent despair; sacred choirs, demoniacal shrieks, acrobatic per-
formances, the chiming of bells, the blasts of trumpets, bray-
ings, lowings, neighings; the crackling fires beneath
cauldrons, heaps of fruits and sweets, shop windows full of
utensils, draperies, arms, jewels, rosaries; the obscene contor-
tions of dancing girls, the convulsions of epileptics, the blows
of brawlers, the flight of thieves pursued in the throng; the
scum of the worst corruptions brought forth from the filthy
alleys of distant towns and cast upon an ignorant and amazed
multitude; clouds of implacable parasites, like horseflies about
cattle, falling upon the compact crowd, incapable of self-
defense; every base temptation for brutal appetites, every fraud
to trick the simple and the stupid, every immodesty was

28. Gabriele D'Annunzio, *Trionfo della morte*, in *Prose di romanzi*, 1:895–96.

exhibited in broad daylight; all mixtures were there, seething
and fermenting around the House of the Virgin.]

This Pandora's box of evils and ills is a magnified portion of Ippolita
herself: her epilepsy and gynecological disturbances. The scene of
mass hysteria to which this passage alludes is the ostensible cause
of Ippolita's hysterical attack, the lower classes of the body politic
seeming to irritate the "lower" functions of the female body. That
hysteria threatens to awaken the "male sacro" that afflicts her,
which is an obstruction of the erotic intercourse between Ippolita
and Giorgio Aurispa: "Se questo male mi prendesse fra le tue
braccia? No, no, io non ti vedrò più, non voglio più vederti"
(*Trionfo,* 920) ["What if this malady were to seize me while I was
in your arms? No, no, I will not see you anymore, I do not wish
to see you anymore"]. Giorgio Aurispa's reading of cause and effect,
however, identifies Ippolita as the cause of mass hysteria; the crowd
is Ippolita's projection: "Forse io vedo il suo sogno. E il suo sogno
ha forse per causa la perturbazione che incomincia nei suoi organi
e che aumenterà sino all'accesso. Non è talvolta un sogno il presagio
d'un morbo covato?" (*Trionfo,* 918) ["Perhaps I see her dream. And
perhaps the cause of her dream is the disturbance that begins in
her organs and will increase until it is an attack. Is not a dream
sometimes the presage of a hidden malady?"]. The crowd and the
woman, linked through their sickness and surrender to physiology,
come to represent the (necessary) underside of Giorgio's erotic
scenarios. Ippolita's dream is but the manifestation of her physiological ills, the body's nightmare of deformation and amputation;
the epileptic attack she observes and fears is a demonic version of
her ecstasy in love. The crowd and the woman are elements of an
erotic discourse that would be alien and antagonistic to the rhetoric
of convalescence in *Il piacere.*

Leaving aside, for the moment, the question of female sickness
in D'Annunzio's novels, I nonetheless propose that the crowd is
tainted by that sickness. Several discourses on sexuality meet and
conflict in *Il piacere,* but the eroticism grounded in female sickness
is absent from this section of the novel. Convalescence itself retains
an erotic element (art as faithful lover, Maria Ferres as *turris eburnea*);
like Augustine's conversion, convalescence is a turning away from
a particular eros, not from eros *tout court.* In the sections of the

novel that sandwich book 2, scenes of locker-room vulgarity in social gatherings (for example, Mount Edgcumbe's pornographic library or the episode concerning Sperelli's ex-lover, who lacks, much to the men's amusement and horror, "la douce barbe feminine" ["the sweet feminine beard"]) alternate with the attempts of Sperelli and Elena to "trasformare in alto sentimento un basso appetito" (*Il piacere*, 268) ["to transform a low appetite into noble sentiment"]. The veils of art and sentiment are rent, Sperelli's eloquence is made to seem a spiel, by contact with such mundane scenes. The eroticism of female sickness with which the crowd is associated might have a similarly demystifying effect on the convalescent's project. The convalescent is the site of an intersection between psychology and physiology; lingering sickness is the ground of a new consciousness, a new interpretation of the body's relation to thought. The crowd would thus represent a physiology the protagonist seeks to avoid, which the convalescent, for his project to be successful, must reinterpret. The convalescent, whose fevers and congestion grant him an alternative vision, explores a different physiology and proposes a different interpretation of the body.

Feminization

Convalescence is a space in-between, a vector that points toward health and away from sickness, a copresence of symptoms of health and sickness. As a commingling of opposites, convalescence becomes the ground for figures of physiological ambiguity, of, one might almost say, physiological monstrosity. Yet at first it seems quite unmonstrous that the convalescent's rebirth should be figured as a return to childhood and innocence:

> Or, la convalescence est comme un retour vers l'enfance. Le convalescent jouit au plus haut degré, comme l'enfant, de la faculté de s'intéresser vivement aux choses, même les plus triviales en apparence. Remontons, s'il se peut, par un effort rétrospectif de l'imagination, vers nos plus jeunes, nos plus matinales impressions, et nous reconnaîtrons qu'elles avaient une singulière parenté avec des impressions si vivement colo-

rées, que nous reçûmes plus tard à la suite d'une maladie physique, pourvu que cette maladie ait laissé pures et intactes nos facultés spirituelles. L'enfant voit tout en *nouveauté;* il est toujours *ivre.* (*Le peintre,* 690)

[Now convalescence is like a return towards childhood. The convalescent, like the child, is possessed in the highest degree of the faculty of keenly interesting himself in things, be they apparently of the most trivial. Let us go back, if we can, by a retrospective effort of the imagination, towards our most youthful, our earliest, impressions, and we will recognize that they had a strange kinship with those brightly coloured impressions which we were later to receive in the aftermath of a physical illness, always provided that that illness had left our spiritual capacities pure and unharmed. The child sees everything in a state of newness; he is always *drunk.* (Mayne, 7–8)]

The vivid perceptions of the child are due to extraordinary receptiveness, to the absence of any hierarchizing faculty; even the most trivial things interest him. Baudelaire's *enfant,* in these lines, calls to mind another ingenuous child who perceives the poetry in particulars, Giovanni Pascoli's *fanciullino.* But as we read on, Baudelaire's child grows away from Pascoli's innocent, for he is subject to a congestion whose nature is uncertain:

Rien ne ressemble plus à ce qu'on appelle l'inspiration, que la joie avec laquelle l'enfant absorbe la forme et la couleur. J'oserai pousser plus loin; j'affirme que l'inspiration a quelque rapport avec la *congestion,* et que toute pensée sublime est accompagnée d'une secousse nerveuse, plus ou moins forte, qui retentit jusque dans le cervelet. L'homme de génie a les nerfs solides; l'enfant les a faibles. (*Le peintre,* 690)

[Nothing more resembles what we call inspiration than the delight with which a child absorbs form and colour. I am prepared to go even further and assert that inspiration has something in common with *congestion,* and that every sublime thought is accompanied by a more or less violent nervous shock which has its repercussion in the very core of the brain. The man of genius has very sound nerves, while those of the child are weak. (Mayne, 8; trans. modified)]

Congestion and nervous shock have turned a bright-eyed innocent into a sickly neurasthenic child who receives shocks similar to those of the pathological man of the crowd's electrified intellect. But a sentence later a different source is suggested for the child's excitation and congestion:

Mais le génie n'est que l'*enfance retrouvée* à volonté, l'enfance douée maintenant, pour s'exprimer, d'organes virils et de l'esprit analytique qui lui permet d'ordonner la somme de matériaux involontairement amassée. (*Le peintre,* 690)

[But genius is nothing more than *childhood recovered* at will— a childhood now equipped for self-expression with manhood's capacities and a power of analysis which enables it to order the mass of raw material which it has involuntarily accumulated. (Mayne, 8)]

In order to read this passage smoothly, one must accept the pressures exerted upon us by the text to identify "organes virils" with "nerfs solides." We are thus constrained to accept the definition of virility as fortitude and forbearance (as indeed Mayne's translation does by rendering "organes virils" not as virile organs but as "manhood's capacities"). But if we resist this pressure and give full rein to the play of meaning, we are confronted with an insinuation of childhood sexuality which would have shocked Pascoli. The physiological ambiguity (if not monstrosity) thus evoked—a sexually mature, fully rational child—is a figure for the convalescent's privileged interpretation of the body's relationship to thought. Is it the "esprit analytique" that interprets a questionably childish body, the "organes virils" that give it expression? A phrase from "Un mangeur d'opium" would seem to confirm this hypothesis: "Le génie n'est que l'enfance nettement formulée, douée, mainten- ant, pour s'exprimer, d'organes virils et puissants" ["Genius is nothing other than childhood clearly formulated, now endowed

with virile and powerful organs with which to express himself"].[29]
An entire narrative unfolds from this image of a child onto whom
have been grafted virile organs "pour s'exprimer." The convalescent
has undergone not only a kind of death and rebirth but a kind of
eviration. The man is reduced to a child, a child who is, however,
fitted with a prosthesis, an instrument of self-expression lacking in
literal childhood. The intimation of castration suggests that the
return to childhood is a euphemism for feminization. Indeed, an
equivalence is established not between "l'homme de génie" and
"l'enfant" but between two states of being, "le génie" and "l'enfance." Thus virile organs are attributed to a feminine "enfance."
Linguistic gender hints at the feminization that occurs, as we shall
see, in the convalescences of Sperelli, des Esseintes, and Nietzsche.
The sharply marked division between sickness and convalescence
introduces a division of the "feminine"; the expulsion of woman
from the scene of convalescence is not the expulsion of her attributes. Indeed, woman is expelled in order that her qualities may be
abstracted and reassigned to the convalescent himself. Baudelaire's
chain of terms for Constantin Guys seems ironclad in masculinity,
but in the subsection "Femmes et filles" of Le peintre we find what
might well be a description of Andrea Sperelli's relationship to the
liquidated crowd:

Ces deux êtres ne pensent pas. Est-il bien sûr même qu'ils
regardent? à moins que, Narcisses de l'imbécillité, ils ne
contemplent la foule comme un fleuve qui leur rend leur
image. En réalité, ils existent bien plutôt pour le plaisir de
l'observateur que pour leur plaisir propre. (Le peintre, 719)

[These two beings have not a single thought in their heads. Is
it even certain that they can see? Unless, like Narcissuses of
imbecility, they are gazing at the crowd as at a river which
reflects their own image. In truth, they exist very much more
for the pleasure of the observer than for their own. (Mayne, 35)]

As in Il piacere, the crowd becomes a body of water that reflects
the image of the observer. The text invites a comparison with

29. Baudelaire, "Un mangeur d'opium," Les paradis artificiels, 1:498.

Baudelaire's convalescent as well, for these two creatures are similarly positioned on the threshold, "à la porte d'un café, s'appuyant aux vitres illuminées par devant et par derrière" (*Le peintre,* 719) ["at a café door, leaning against the windows lit from within and without" (Mayne, 35; trans. modified)]. Their relationship to the crowd thus constitutes a countertext to Monsieur Guys's contemplation: "Derrière la vitre d'un café, un convalescent, contemplant la foule avec jouissance, se mêle par la pensée." Moreover, in this subsection devoted to describing female types "jusqu'à la *foemina simplex,*" a male figure is introduced only in this paragraph. These "êtres" are a "fille de théâtre" and her male companion, yet the masculine plural pronouns absorb and efface the feminine presence. The masculinization of the woman is further underscored by her unwomanly activity: "Comme son joli compagnon, elle a tout l'orifice de sa petite bouche occupé par un cigare disproportionné" (*Le peintre,* 719) ["Like her dainty companion, she has an enormous cigar entirely filling the aperture of her tiny mouth" (Mayne, 35)]. That smoking is considered unwomanly is confirmed by Baudelaire's description of the *foemina simplex:* "Elles se montrent prostrées dans les attitudes désesperées d'ennui, dans des indolences d'estaminet, d'un cynisme masculin, fumant des cigarettes pour tuer le temps" (*Le peintre,* 721) ["They display themselves in hopeless attitudes of boredom, in bouts of tap-room apathy, almost masculine in their cynicism, killing time with cigarettes" (Mayne, 37; trans. modified)]. The commingling of masculine and feminine in contemplating the crowd could represent merely the inability of the lower-class "êtres" to achieve the upper-class convalescent's level of consciousness. Yet if we return now to our monstrous child, we discover that he is not so dissimilar from these "Narcisses de l'imbécillité":

C'est à cette curiosité profonde et joyeuse qu'il faut attribuer l'oeil fixe et animalement extatique des enfants devant le *nouveau,* quel qu'il soit, visage ou paysage, lumière, dorure, couleurs, étoffes chatoyantes, enchantements de la beauté embellie par la toilette. (*Le peintre,* 690)

[It is by this deep and joyful curiosity that we may explain the fixed and animally ecstatic gaze of a child confronted with something new, whatever it be, whether a face or a landscape, gilding, colours, shimmering stuffs, or the magic of physical beauty assisted by cosmetic art. (Mayne, 8)]

At this point, the rereader of Baudelaire might assume that the phrase "la beauté embellie par la toilette" is an allusion to the later subsection "L'éloge du maquillage" in which Baudelaire argues against the commonplace that "la nature embellit la beauté" ["nature beautifies beauty"]. Encouraged by the "étoffes chatoyantes," we might, then, expect the figure of a woman to appear, for it is the woman who profits from the art of cosmetics in Baudelaire's essay. But no; our virile child contemplates a version of himself:

Un de mes amis me disait un jour qu'étant fort petit, il assistait à la toilette de son père, et qu'alors il contemplait, avec une stupeur mêlée de délices, les muscles des bras, les dégradations de couleurs de la peau nuancée de rose et de jaune, et le réseau bleuâtre des veines. Le tableau de la vie extérieure le pénétrait déjà de respect et s'emparait de son cerveau. Déjà la forme l'obsédait et le possédait. (*Le peintre,* 690–91)

[A friend of mine once told me that when he was quite a small child, he used to be present when his father dressed in the mornings, and that it was with a mixture of amazement and delight that he used to study the muscles of his arms, the gradual transitions of pink and yellow in his skin, and the bluish network of his veins. The picture of external life was already filling him with awe and taking hold of his brain. He was already being obsessed and possessed by form. (Mayne, 8)]

Thus, a vision of male beauty where the text teased us to expect a female one, masculine pronouns referring to the woman who contemplates her image in the riverlike crowd, suggest a tension between masculinization and femininization. The child seems to contemplate a version of himself, yet that contemplation emphasizes his femininity. Not only is the father's activity marked as womanly by the text, but the language of the mind's activity is borrowed from that of sexuality. The language of the quoted passage is not that of the mind's penetration into things, but of its receptivity and invasion. The child, grammatical object of the object he observes ("le pénétrait," "s'emparait de son cerveau," "l'obsédait et le possédait"), is penetrated and possessed by the image of the father. As Leo Bersani has suggested in his reading of the *Journaux intimes,* psychic penetrability is figurally related to sexual penetrability.[30]

Such psychic penetrability is one of Sperelli's symptoms:

> A poco a poco, in quegli ozii intenti e raccolti, il suo spirito si stendeva, si svolgeva, si dispiegava, si sollevava dolcemente come l'erba premuta in su' sentieri; diveniva infine verace, ingenuo, originale, libero, aperto alla pura conoscenza, disposto alla pura contemplazione; attirava in sè le cose, le concepiva come modalità del suo proprio essere, come forme della sua propria esistenza; si sentiva infine penetrato dalla verità che proclama l'Oupanischad dei Veda: "Hae omnes creaturae in totum ego sum, et praeter me aliud ens non est." (*Il piacere,* 136)

> [Little by little, in this silent and intent idleness, his spirit expanded, unwound, uncoiled, lifted itself gently like grass trodden underfoot on the path; it became truthful, ingenuous, original, free, open to pure knowledge, ready for pure contemplation. It drew things into itself, conceived of them as modalities of its own being, as forms of its existence. He felt himself penetrated by the truth of the Veda Upanishad: "Hae omnes creaturae in totum ego sum, et praeter me aliud ens non est."]

The first, absorbent phase of convalescence precedes, in both Baudelaire and D'Annunzio, a second phase in which all that has been so absorbed will be expressed in the form of Guys's sketches and Sperelli's poems. In *Il piacere* this first phase is similarly described as a return to childhood; in the very paragraph in which this topos is introduced, a father appears:

30. See Leo Bersani, *Baudelaire and Freud* (Berkeley: University of California Press, 1977), 12.

Il convalescente rinveniva sensazioni obliate della puerizia, quell'impression di freschezza che dànno al sangue puerile gli aliti del vento salso, quegli inesprimibili effetti che fanno le luci, le ombre, i colori, gli odori delle acque su l'anima vergine. Il mare non soltanto era per lui una delizia degli occhi, ma era una perenne onda di pace a cui si abbeveravano i suoi pensieri, una magica fonte di giovinezza in cui il suo corpo riprendeva la salute e il suo spirito la nobiltà. Il mare aveva per lui l'attrazion misteriosa d'una patria, ed egli vi si abbandonava con un confidenza filiale, come un figliuol debole nelle braccia d'un padre onnipossente. E ne riceveva conforto; poiché nessuno mai ha confidato il suo dolore, il suo desiderio, il suo sogno al mare invano. (*Il piacere*, 139–40)

[The convalescent rediscovered forgotten sensations of his childhood, that impression of freshness that the salt breeze gives to young blood, those indescribable effects produced by the lights, shadows, colors and smells of the sea on the virgin soul. The sea was not only a delight to his eyes, but also a perennial wave of peace in which his thoughts drank deep, a magic fountain of youth in which his body regained health and his spirit, nobility. The sea had for him the mysterious attraction of a fatherland, and he abandoned himself to it with filial trust, like a feeble son in the arms of an omnipotent father. And he received comfort; for no one has ever confided his pain, his desire or his dream to the sea in vain.]

To be sure, the corporeality of the Baudelairean father—all muscles, veins, and shimmering skin—is absent here, the D'Annunzian father assuming divine proportions and insubstantiality. Yet the text creates a similar ambiguity of expectations; this babe in arms is held not by a mother (as the play on *mare/madre* might suggest) but by a father whose name is grammatically feminine. Of itself, such a detail might be insignificant were it not exploited in Italian politico-patriotic parlance by the term *madrepatria,* a hermaphroditic term that D'Annunzio himself employs in his later speeches at Fiume. The sea as mother-fatherland not only comforts but subjugates, for one paragraph later we find the convalescent/child yoked and crushed by its powers. Like the Baudelairean father, it overwhelms and possesses the observer:

> In certe ore il convalescente, sotto l'assiduo dominio d'una tal virtù, sotto l'assiduo giogo di un tal fascino, provava una specie di smarrimento e quasi di sbigottimento, come se quel dominio e quel giogo fossero per la sua debolezza insostenibili. (*Il piacere,* 140)

> [At times, under the continuous domination of such an influence, under the assiduous yoke of such fascination, the convalescent felt a sort of bewilderment and almost fear, as though both the domination and yoke were unbearable to his weakness.]

The convalescent's earlier openness to the contemplation of the sea is intensified to a feeling of total domination. The suggestion of feminization in Sperelli's convalescence remains, however, faint; in order to strengthen it we must make yet another detour. Tension between masculinization and feminization in the scene of convalescence resonates more loudly when we add Huysmans's *A rebours* to the texts considered.

Jean Des Esseintes, too, moves to a liminal position in order to indulge in a long (and ultimately failed) convalescence. No *homme des foules,* the ailing protagonist flees contact with the crowd to establish himself in a place not too near yet not too far from the city:

> En songeant à la nouvelle existence qu'il voulait organiser, il éprouvait une allégresse d'autant plus vive qu'il se voyait retiré assez loin déjà, sur la berge, pour que le flot de Paris ne l'atteignit plus et assez près cependant pour que cette proximité de la capitale le confirmât dans sa solitude.

> [Thinking of the new existence he was going to fashion for himself, he felt a glow of pleasure at the idea that here he would be too far out for the tidal wave of Parisian life to reach

him, and yet near enough for the proximity of the capital to strengthen him in his solitude.][31]

In taking leave of the city he takes leave of the debauchery that contributed to his frightful state of health; an expulsion of woman from his existence coincides with his retirement into seclusion. We need not insinuate such an expulsion into the text; it is marked clamorously and glamorously by a "repas de deuil," a sort of symphony in black which commemorates the death of his virility: "Le dîner de faire-part d'une virilité momentanément morte, était-il écrit sur les lettres d'invitations semblables à celles des enterrements" (A rebours, 95) ["On the invitations, which were similar to those sent out before more solemn obsequies, this dinner was described as a funeral banquet in memory of the host's virility, lately but only temporarily deceased" (Baldick, 27)]. His virility buried—and virility here refers explicitly to sexual potency—Des Esseintes can devote himself to aesthetic matters. We may, at this point, add to the accumulation of Baudelairean bons mots which Huysmans's text actualizes, for in the Journaux intimes Baudelaire vividly characterizes the relationship between sexual potency and the arts: "Plus l'homme cultive les arts, moins il bande" ["The more man cultivates the arts, the fewer erections he has"].[32] Des Esseintes seems, moreover, to have been destined for just such a burial not only by his funereal childhood but by his heredity: "La décadence de cette ancienne maison avait, sans nul doute, suivi regulièrement son cours; l'effémination des mâles était allée en s'accentuant; comme pour achever l'oeuvre des âges, les des Esseintes marièrent, pendant deux siècles, leurs enfants entre eux, usant leur reste de vigueur dans les unions consanguines" (A rebours, 80). ["The degeneration of this ancient house had clearly followed a regular course, with the men becoming progressively less manly; and over the last two hundred years, as if to complete the ruinous process, the Des Esseintes had taken to intermarrying among themselves, thus using up what little vigour they had left" (Baldick,

31. Huysmans, A rebours, ed. Fumaroli, 88, Against Nature, trans. Baldick, 24, hereafter cited parenthetically in the text.
32. Baudelaire, "Mon coeur mis à nu," in Journaux intimes, in Oeuvres complètes, 1:702.

17)]. The decadent topoi of a genetically exhausted nobility and the feminization of men ("L'homme s'affine, se féminise, se divinise") merge in Huysmans as they did in Lombroso, degeneration becoming degenderation. Des Esseintes's feminization is further underscored by his nocturnal habit. Though he rejects certain seductive colors from his decorator's scheme ("Il n'y avait pas à songer davantage aux saumons, aux maïs et aux roses dont les efféminations contrarieraient les pensées de l'isolement" [*A rebours*, 96] ["Nor was there any point in thinking of such delicate tints as salmon pink, maize, and rose; for their very effeminacy would run counter to his ideas of complete isolation" (Baldick, 29)]), his choice of the night as most appropriate to his hours of activity ("Il ne vivait guère que la nuit [*A rebours*, 95] ["He lived most of his life at night" (Baldick, 28)]) is a return to childhood and to his mother's preference for heavily curtained dusk: "Elle s'absorbait de nouveau dans la nuit factice dont les épais rideaux des croisées enveloppaient la chambre" (*A rebours*, 81–82) ["She sank back again into the artificial night which the heavy curtains drawn across the windows created in her bedroom" (Baldick, 19)]. Interestingly, the night is one of the few "real" elements accepted by this proponent of artificiality: his mother's was an artificial night; his is a natural one. Sperelli returns to a mother nature, Des Esseintes to a naturalized mother artificiality.

While Des Esseintes's eviration is the result of illness—generic syphilis coupled with a severe *dégoût du réel*, the *réel* including women and food—Sperelli's eviration *is* the illness. A figurative death of virility precedes and necessitates his convalescence. The "mortale ferita" ["mortal wound"] from which Sperelli langorously recovers is inflicted in a duel with Gianetto Rutolo, a minor character who functions only as Sperelli's rival for the attentions of another minor character, Donna Ippolita. The literal wound inflicted in this duel seems not to be quite as fatal as its consequences would suggest. It is a "ferita toracica, al quarto spazio intercostale destro, penetrante in cavità, con lesione superficiale del polmone" (*Il piacere*, 133) ["wound penetrating the thorax through the fourth intercostal space on the right side with superficial wound of the lung"]. One is tempted to observe, as T. S. Eliot did of Hamlet, that the emotion expressed ("mortale ferita") is in excess of the facts as they appear. The literal wound is, of course, not the point; the effect is less important than the cause, for the duel is fought not with pistols, as might be expected in a late nineteenth-century novel, but with swords. We need not have recourse to vulgar Freudian symbolism in order to suggest that swords second the phallus, for a much stronger argument is supplied by Ariostean and Tassian versions and subversions of the phallic valence of swords and dueling.[33] In the code of those chivalric romances, loss of a duel is a loss of power as well as potency; the swordless warrior is effeminate (it is for this reason that Rinaldo mirrors himself in a *scudo*, a womanly arm). The very anachronism of a duel with swords underscores its link with the duels of romance and marks it as phallic combat. Sperelli, then, loses the duel, lays down the sword. Death of desire is the result: "Egli riposava, poiché non desiderava più. Il desiderio aveva abbandonato il suo regno" (*Il piacere*, 137) ["He rested, for he no longer desired. Desire had abandoned its reign"]. Croce and Salinari's allusions to the gardens of Alcina and Armida thus begin to seem pertinent, though by hypallage, for the characteristics of Sperelli the convalescent are attributed to D'Annunzio the author. Sperelli might indeed be said to be held in thrall by Donna Maria, just as Rinaldo and Ruggiero were held by Armida and Alcina. Artistic creation takes place in just such gardens, for eviration marks the entrance into convalescence as the artist's rite of passage. Salinari and Croce posit precisely the opposite: the artist's rite of passage occurs when he takes up the sword and leaves the garden. Their criticism is a counterargument rather than a reading of the text, an assertion of an opposing ideology rather than a critique of the text's ideology.

But doesn't the image of a sorceress's garden as the locus of convalescence conflict with the expulsion of woman I have described? Is not convalescence a liberation from the dandy's dalliance with women and thus in some sense an escape from the siren song? It is and it is not. The several rhetorics employed to characterize convalescence—that of conversion, that of a return to childhood, and that of feminization—intertwine in a complex and puzzling way. Sperelli's convalescence is described in the terms of Christian conversion:

33. See John C. McLucas, "Ariosto and the Androgyne: Symmetries of Sex in the *Orlando Furioso*" (Ph.D. diss., Yale University, 1983).

Dopo la mortale ferita, dopo una specie di lunga e lenta agonia, Andrea Sperelli ora a poco a poco rinasceva, quasi con un altro corpo e con un altro spirito, come un uomo nuovo, come una creatura uscita da un fresco bagno letèo, immemore e vacua. (*Il piacere*, 135)

[After the mortal wound, after a sort of long, slow agony, Andrea Sperelli was little by little reborn, as though with an other body and with an other spirit, like a new man, like a creature who has emerged from a cool Lethean bath, empty and without memory.]

Sperelli's rebirth and entrance into an earthly paradise recalls the cleansing of Dante the pilgrim as he crosses the river Lethe, leaves Purgatory and ascends to Paradise. The old man is taken off, the new put on, and both body and soul are renewed. The convalescent's conversion marks not a scission between mind and body but the emergence of a new consciousness that can only be described in relation to this "altro corpo":

Comprende egli che la sua vita reale è quella, dirò così, non vissuta da lui; è il complesso delle sensazioni involontarie, spontanee, inconscienti, istintive; è l'attività armoniosa e misteriosa della vegetazione animale; è l'impercettibile sviluppo di tutte le metamorfosi e di tutte le rinnovellazioni. Quella vita appunto in lui compie i miracoli della convalescenza: richiude le piaghe, ripara le perdite, riallaccia le trame infrante, rammenda i tessuti lacerati, ristaura i congegni degli organi, rinfonde nelle vene la ricchezza del sangue, riannoda su gli occhi la benda dell'amore, rintreccia d'intorno al capo la corona de' sogni, riaccende nel cuore la fiamma della speranza, riapre le ali alle chimere della fantasia. (*Il piacere*, 135)

[He understands that his real life is the one, I will say it thus, not lived by him. It is the complex of involuntary, spontaneous, unconscious, instinctive sensations. It is the harmonious and mysterious activity of animal vegetation, the imperceptible development of all metamorphoses and all renewals. Precisely that life performs the miracles of convalescence: it heals wounds, makes up for losses, reweaves the broken woof, mends lacerated tissues, restores the tissue of the organs, reinfuses the veins with rich blood, reknots the blindfold of love about the eyes, replaits the crown of dreams about the head, reignites the flame of hope within the heart, reopens the wings of the chimera of the imagination.]

"L'altro corpo" thus seems to be the wounded body, whose imperceptible sensations are perceived in the state of convalescence; the "true" life is that which makes its way through tissues, organs, and blood and mounts toward the mind's activity: dreams, hope, imagination. But could it be that this "altro corpo" is also the "corpo dell'altro," the body of the Other? The new body, which is the consequence of eviration and which desires no longer, is, I have suggested, characterized as feminine. Thus we might say that the "old woman" is expelled in order that the "new woman" might be put on, that the converted convalescent might assume a feminine guise. The mind's activity is described in terms of corporeal activity marked as feminine; the convalescent's mind is penetrated and invaded so that it might give birth to verse:

Gli pareva che le rime, uscenti a mano a mano dal suo cervello, avessero un sapor nuovo. La consonanza gli veniva spontanea, senza ch'ei la cercasse; e i pensieri gli nascevano rimati. . . . La strofe alla fine gli usciva intera e precisa. . . . tutto il sonetto viveva e respirava come un organismo indipendente, nell'unità. (*Il piacere,* 151–52)

[It seemed to him that the rhymes, emerging gradually from his brain, had a new taste. Consonance came to him spontaneously and with no effort on his part; thoughts were born in rhymes. . . . Finally the verse emerged from him whole and precise. . . . the entire sonnet lived and breathed like an independent creature, in unity.]

That the poet's production should be couched in the terms of human reproduction may seem far from startling, quite commonplace; such a conception relies in fact upon the notion that "a man becomes a woman when he writes." Probably the most eloquent statement of this ideologeme is to be found in Gaston Bachelard's *Poetics of Reverie,* where, with the help of Jung, he theorizes the psychology of poetic creation: "Reverie is under the sign of the *anima.* When the reverie is truly profound, the being who comes to dream within us is our *anima.*"[34] Bachelard swiftly links this notion of poetic reverie to that of the androgyny of the poet's mind; the encounter of animus and anima thus constitutes the ground and essence of poetry. Jung and Bachelard are, of course, not alone in proposing that great minds are androgynous. Coleridge and Virginia Woolf preceded them, and D'Annunzio, too, seems to concur. Andrea Sperelli's muse, Maria Ferres, is an androgynous figure:

> Era una voce ambigua, direi quasi bisessuale, duplice, andro-
> ginica; di due timbri. Il timbro maschile, basso e un poco
> velato, s'ammorbidiva, si chiariva, s'infemminiva talvolta con
> passaggi così armoniosi che l'orecchio dell' uditore n'aveva
> sorpresa e diletto a un tempo e perplessità. (*Il piacere,* 169)

> [It was an ambiguous voice, I would almost say bisexual,
> double, androgynous; of two timbres. The masculine timbre,
> low and slightly veiled, would soften, grow brighter and more
> feminine at times with such harmonious transitions that the
> ear of the listener would catch in it both delight and
> perplexity.]

The double synonymic dittology of this passage (bisessuale/androgi-nica, duplice/di due timbri) is iconic of the double nature of Maria's voice. As we shall see, it is not coincidental that her voice, rather than her person, is described as androgynous. It is the voice of a muse figure, after all, which would be emphasized, but it is also true that a description of her person as androgynous would evoke the androgyne's material counterpart, the hermaphrodite, which represents not a spiritual ideal but physiological monstrosity. The very mention of androgyny seems to evoke its carnival freak cousin:

---

34. Gaston Bachelard, *The Poetics of Reverie: Childhood, Language and the Cosmos,* trans. Daniel Russell (Boston: Beacon, 1969), 62, hereafter cited in the text; trans. of *La poétique de la rêverie* (Paris: Presses Universitaires de France, 1960).

Andrea Sperelli's published work is titled *La favola d'ermafrodito*
[*The Tale of the Hermaphrodite*]. The spiritual configuration is accompanied by its corporeal transfiguration. The coupling of androgyne
and hermaphrodite, appearing in the context of the convalescent's
exploration of the body's relationship to thought, disturbs the
pacific notion of a spiritual union of masculine and feminine.

As a seemingly unproblematic solution to the riddle of "how a man
becomes a woman when he writes," androgyny is a solution riddled
with problems. Frequently offered as a rebuttal to feminist criticism,
the androgyne argument is truly two-faced. While denying the validity and necessity of feminist criticism, except as a sociological approach, in the name of a genderless art or philosophy, at the same
moment it excludes women from the production of art and philosophy. Feminist criticism is described as talking about physiological
distinctions that have no place in the realm of the abstract qualities
"masculine" and "feminine." In fact the *ad feminam* argument usually
employed degrades the opponent's argument by claiming that it
speaks of "lower" matters—skirts and pants (under which euphe-
misms lie the genitals)—and thereby insists upon a sexual difference
that exists in a court of law but not in art: "In everyday life, the words
'man' and 'woman'—dresses and pants—are sufficient designations.
But in the muted life of the subconscious, in the retiring life of a
solitary dreamer, peremptory designations lose their authority. The
words *animus* and *anima* have been chosen to soften the sexual designations and escape the simplicity of birth certificate classifications"
(Bachelard, 66). Once we have "escaped" that simplicity, however,
we discover another hitch in the notion of androgyny as the poetic
condition. If androgyny consists in the man of a commingling of his
dominant animus with the anima of Bachelard's reverie, what then
of the woman whose anima is already dominant? This problem evokes
what Luce Irigaray has called "the blind spot of an ancient dream of
symmetry": the theoretical model applied to the male subject begins
to grind its gears when transferred to the female subject upon which
it relies as otherness.[35] Bachelard, not unaware of this problem, opts
for a nonsymmetrical solution:

35. See Luce Irigaray, *Speculum of the Other Woman*, trans. Gillian C. Gill
(Ithaca: Cornell University Press, 1985), trans. of *Speculum de l'autre femme* (Paris:
Minuit, 1974).

> On the other hand, by agreeing to the reference to two psychological instances, *anima* and *animus,* in order to classify our reflections on the essential femininity of any deep reverie, we are, we believe, protecting ourselves from an objection. One could, in fact, object—by following the automatism from which so many philosophical dialectics suffer—that if the man centered on the *animus* dreams the reverie in *anima,* the woman centered on the *anima* should dream in *animus.* Doubtless, the tension of civilization is presently such that "feminism" commonly reinforces the *animus* of the woman... It has been repeated often enough that feminism ruins femininity. But once again, if one wishes to give reverie its fundamental character, if he wishes to take it as a state, a present state which has no need for the scaffolding of *projects,* it is necessary to recognize that reverie liberates any dreamer, man or woman, from the world of demands. . . . In a pure reverie which returns the dreamer to his tranquil solitude, every human being, man or woman, finds his repose in the *anima* of the depths, by descending, ever descending "the slope of reverie." (Bachelard, 63)

The state of reverie is thus, for man and woman alike, found in the anima. By opting for the nonsymmetrical solution, Bachelard aims to shore up his ontology of androgyny, of the anima (within the man), as the essence of poetry. In consequence, however, it becomes clear that androgyny as the poetic condition cannot exist for the woman, for where is the animus that would supply the "andro"? In poetic reverie, she is double anima. The presence of the animus in the woman destroys (Bachelard and Jung concur) the feminine in her; animus and anima are antagonistic forces, which produce animosity.[36] Far from becoming a poet, the woman cannot even

36. Though "animosity" characterizes the relationship of animus to anima in both male and female subjects, the combination woman-animus produces greater enmity: "Whereas the cloud of 'animosity' surrounding the man is composed chiefly of sentimentality and resentment, in woman it expresses itself in the form of opinionated views, interpretations, insinuations, and misconstructions, which all have the purpose (sometimes attained) of severing the relation between two human beings." C. G. Jung, "The Synygy: Anima and Animus," in *Aion: Researches into the Phenomenology of the Self,* trans. R. F. C. Hull, Bollingen Series 20 (Princeton: Princeton University Press, 1968), 9:2, 16.

speak, for Bachelard describes immersion in the anima as a state that drowns the dreamer: "Reading, ever reading, the sweet passion of the *anima*. But when, after having read everything, one sets before himself the task of making a book out of reveries, it is the *animus* which is in the harness" (Bachelard, 65). The woman's animus could conceivably return at this moment, but Bachelard no longer concerns himself with the relationship of the woman to reverie. Without the androgynous mixture of masculine and feminine, one cannot, it seems, even speak. Bachelard's persistent efforts to idealize sexual difference as animus and anima, in order "not to fall victim to simplistic physiological designation" (Bachelard, 66), rely not on the harmonious resolution of sexual difference but on the elimination of the marked term, woman, which reminds us that such difference exists.[37] She is, once again, silenced, emptied of her attributes so that they may be put on by the male poet. The idealizing project would take place in her absence, but "vulgar" physiology haunts its steps; androgyny must, if it is to attain philosophical purity, be cleansed of this shadowy presence.

Physiology haunts the androgyne's foot-less steps in the very language employed to express the merging of masculine and feminine; androgyny as a spiritual configuration finds expression in the language that describes the body. Sperelli's poetic production, as I have noted, is described as giving birth. Baudelaire, in "Un mangeur d'opium," utilizes the childhood of Thomas de Quincey as an occasion to promote androgyny as the ground of genius:

L'homme qui, dès le commencement, a été longtemps baigné dans la molle atmosphère de la femme, dans l'odeur de ses mains, de son sein, de ses genoux, de sa chevelure, de ses vêtements souples et flottants,

37. The notion of androgyny as just such a pacific "resolution" permeates the criticism of decadent texts. Michel Lemaire, for example, writes: "But dandyism represents an attempt to fuse into a single, superior being the principles that divide man and the world: active and passive, *yang* and *yin*, male and female, *animus* and *anima*, sadism and masochism. . . . Does this androgyne not refer to a golden age, before the fall into duality and sin, another world in which the multiplicity of things would participate in the happiness of unity?" See Michel Lemaire, *Le dandysme de Baudelaire à Mallarmé* (Paris: Klincksieck, 1978), 60.

> Dulce balneum suavibus
> Unguentatum odoribus,

y a contracté une délicatesse d'épiderme et une distinction
d'accent, une espèce d'androgynéité, sans lesquelles le génie
le plus âpre et le plus viril reste, relativement à la perfection
dans l'art, un être incomplet.[38]

[The man who, from the beginning, has long been bathed in
the soft atmosphere of woman, in the odor of her hands, her
breast, her knees, her hair, her supple and flowing clothes
> Dulce balneum suavibus
> Unguentatum odoribus,

has contracted an epidermal delicacy and a distinction of
accent, a sort of androgyny without which the most severe
and virile genius remains, in relation to perfection in art, an
incomplete being.]

The womanly atmosphere in which genius is bathed is the fragrance
of dismembered body parts—hands, breast, knees, hair—whose
enumeration overpowers their "odeur." It is proximity to female
physicality rather than, say, listening to women's conversation,
which completes genius and constitutes androgyny. Bachelard,
too, stumbles upon a body at the very beginning of his reveries on
the gender of words, a body whose monstrosity is doubled by a
mixture of masculine and feminine: "Sometimes the grammatical
act which gives a feminine to a being glorified in the masculine is
pure clumsiness. The centaur is, of course, the prestigious ideal of
a horseman who knows full well that he will never be unseated. But
what might the centauress be? Who can dream of the centauress?"
(Bachelard, 31). Bachelard finds comfort in botany when he discovers that *centaurée* is the name of a flower which "cures torn flesh,"
but the visual image evoked by the mention of a centauress still
irks him and he adds an apologetic footnote: "The word 'centauress'
must be pardoned because Rimbaud could see 'the heights where
seraphic centauresses evolve among the avalanches' (*Les illuminations,* 'Villes'). It is essential, however, to refrain from imagining
them galloping across the plains" (Bachelard, 31). It is essential,

38. Baudelaire, "Un mangeur d'opium," 1:499.

in other words, that the physical realization of the mixture of masculine and feminine not be imagined.[39] The masculine centaur was not presented as a monstrous creature but as "the prestigious ideal of a horseman"; it is the addition of the feminine which brings forth monstrosity. Such an image, for Bachelard, does not belong to the realm of the poetic. But the argument for spiritual androgyny seems to evoke precisely these sorts of images, not in the reader's private reverie but in the texts themselves. The copresence of the androgyne and the hermaphrodite in book 2 of *Il piacere* may stand as an emblem of this phenomenon, for this book is crowded with figures of physiological monstrosity. Sperelli's prized publication, *La favola d'ermafrodito* includes a "Coro dei centauri, delle Sirene e delle Sfingi" ["Chorus of Centaurs, Sirens, and Sphinxes"], and verses spoken by a chimera are cited in the text. In a feverish nightmare, Sperelli interprets storm clouds as "simile ad una zuffa di centauri" ["similar to a battle of centaurs"], as "mostri azzuffati" ["battling monsters"]. Harpies appear to him on the tree of knowledge. Androgyny as a spiritual principle is haunted by the monstrosity of the hermaphrodite; the metonymic chain produced by that hermaphrodite (here, the protagonist's text) is made up of a series of monsters, the majority of which are considered female. Harpies, sphinxes, and sirens are part woman, part animal; the chimera, part lion, part goat, part dragon, is considered a she-monster. References to these monsters appear precisely in the scene of convalescence in which the male protagonist is feminized; they seem to mirror his own condition. Part woman, part animal, they are the demonic versions of the convalescent as part woman part man. If the "altro spirito" the convalescent experiences is androgynous, then the "altro corpo" might be imagined (Bachelard would shudder in horror) as the body of a woman with the head of a man.

Ventriloquism

Des Esseintes, whom we left unpacking his collections of books, paintings, and memories in his new residence, comes closest to

39. Carolyn Heilbrun, in her *Toward a Recognition of Androgyny* (New York: Alfred A. Knopf, 1973), xxi, voiced a similar concern: "One danger perhaps

imagining the convalescent's "altro corpo." Among his memories are two episodes of particular interest, the first that of Miss Urania. Having jogged his memory with a purple bonbon, which contained "une goutte d'essence feminine" ["a drop of female essence"], Des Esseintes reinvisions his encounter with a muscular American acrobat. Inversion is his fantasy:

> Peu à peu, en même temps qu'il l'observait, de singulières conceptions naquirent; à mesure qu'il admirait sa souplesse et sa force, il voyait un artificiel changement de sexe se produire en elle; ses singeries gracieuses, ses mièvreries de femelle s'effaçaient de plus en plus, tandis que se développaient, à leur place, les charmes agiles et puissantes d'un mâle; en un mot, après avoir tout d'abord été femme, puis, après avoir hesité, après avoir avoisiné l'androgyne, elle semblait se résoudre, se préciser, devenir complètement un homme. (*A rebours,* 210–11)

> [Little by little, as he watched her, curious fancies took shape in his mind. The more he admired her suppleness and strength, the more he thought he saw an artificial change of sex operating in her; her mincing movements and feminine affectations became ever less obtrusive, and in their place there developed the agile, vigorous charms of a male. In short, after being a woman to begin with, then hesitating in a condition verging on the androgynous, she seemed to have made up her mind and become an integral, unmistakable man. (Baldick, 111)]

Metamorphosis is specular; while the woman becomes a man, Des Esseintes suffers a sex change: "Il en vint a éprouver, de son côté, l'impression que lui-même se féminisait" (*A rebours,* 211) ["He got to the point of imagining that he for his part was turning female" (Baldick, 111)]. This metamorphosis is not a ground for poetic pyrotechnics on Huysmans's part but seems at first to be an occasion to *épater le bourgeois* by a shocking perversion: a *dominatrix* and an

remains: that androgyny, an ideal, might be confused with hermaphroditism, an anomalous physical condition."

effeminate man. Des Esseintes, aroused by this "échange de sexe," is crushed when his fantasy is deflated by reality: "La transmutation des idées masculines dans son corps de femme n'existait pas" (*A rebours*, 212) ["No transmutation of masculine ideas into her feminine person had occurred" (Baldick, 112)]. Miss Urania turns out to be just another ordinary woman.

But Miss Urania is *not* just another ordinary woman; this *dominatrix* bears the name of one of the muses, and the "échange de sexe" is Des Esseintes—the critic's first attempt at poetic creation. The inversion of sexual roles is also an inversion of poetic roles; if the female muse's traditional role is to inspire the male poet, here it is the male aesthete who would inspire the muse, breathe masculine thoughts into her. His failure to do so generates the subsequent episode in which success is grotesquely attained.

Images of other mistresses follow that of Miss Urania, but Des Esseintes pauses at the memory of a nameless woman "dont la monstruosité l'avait tant satisfait pendant des mois" (*A rebours*, 213) ["whose monstrous speciality had given him months of wonderful satisfaction" (Baldick, 113)]. She is a sideshow ventriloquist, whose monstrous talent Des Esseintes is quick to exploit. Intrigued by the erotic potential of such a gift, Des Esseintes has her memorize a script that triples her monstrosity: the dialogue between the Chimera and the Sphinx from Flaubert's *Tentation de Saint Antoine.* Marble and terracotta statuettes representing the beasts are placed in the bedchamber for the occasion; then, while the ventriloquist projects the carefully rehearsed dialogue into the stone figures, Des Esseintes makes love to her. Through this ploy, Des Esseintes does indeed succeed in "transmuting masculine thoughts into a female body," for while the voice, the material support, is that of the unnamed woman, the words are those of Flaubert. The result of this transmutation is quite literally monstrous, for speech thus seems to originate in the hybrid creatures. His attempt to invert poetic roles had been a dismal failure with Miss Urania; now he succeeds vicariously by substituting a stronger poetic voice for his own. Rather than inspiring his own thoughts into the woman, he inspires the words of a beloved author into her. Indeed, in a further doubling Flaubert too appears to be a ventriloquist; just as the woman projects her voice into and through the statuettes, so Flaubert projects his poetic voice into and through the woman's body.

For Des Esseintes, this coupling of Flaubert and the woman's body is a source of erotic titillation, but for the reader it is suggestive in another sense: ventriloquism, etymologically speech of the stomach or body, may describe the feminized convalescent's relationship to his "altro corpo" and thus may offer another solution to the riddle of how a man becomes a woman when he writes. As Baudelaire and D'Annunzio's choice of androgyny as the poetic state suggests, the convalescent's feminization is not total but a mixture of masculine and feminine. Total feminization would plunge the convalescent into silence or, as we shall see in Chapter 3, lead him to even more brutal forms of death. What is monstrous about this particular mixture is that its constituent parts are still identifiable: the convalescent does not relinquish his voice. Indeed, projected into and through "his" evirated/feminized body—the woman's body—it becomes a poetic voice. The relationship between the body and thought which the convalescent proposes is thus figured as a male voice whose "idées masculines" issue from and by means of the woman's body.

The connection between aesthetic discourse and the woman's body is, of course, dauntingly broad and by no means limited to decadent texts. The scene of ventriloquism in *A rebours* brings to mind a ventriloquist performance of the Enlightenment, Diderot's *Bijoux indiscrets.* There the *ventre* of ventriloquism is taken quite literally, for the speakers of that text are the vaginas of the harem. Though urged to speak of their erotic adventures, the vaginas are also well versed in aesthetics and hold forth at length upon literary and theatrical matters. Diderot himself might be said to be the ventriloquist in this case, projecting his narrative voice into and through the vaginas, for the woman's body here serves as material support for Diderot's discourse on aesthetics. But what is specific to decadent texts—and in particular, to the scene of convalescence—is that the speaker himself is dressed in a feminized body. Woman is expelled from the scene of convalescence precisely in order that the convalescent might occupy her body, might speak from her body.

Des Esseintes the convalescent-aesthete does not in fact speak through the woman's body. He is not a ventriloquist because he is not an artist, and ventriloquism provides him with little more than a means to excite his failing organs. But just as Huysmans has supplied bibliography for the decadents, so does his text offer us a metalanguage with which to analyze the convalescent narratives of decadent texts. The discourses of Constantin Guys, of Andrea Sperelli, and of Nietzsche in his preface to *The Gay Science* all pass through the woman's body. All three are ventriloquists, though the forms and results of their ventriloquism differ. For Constantin Guys, occupation of the woman's body allows a displacement of virility to a prosthetic "organe viril," which, however, expresses itself through the *mundus muliebris*. For Sperelli, the failed poet, occupation of the woman's body for initially poetic ends leads to ventriloquism as a form of seduction. For Nietzsche, the convalescent occupies the woman's body in order to avoid seduction, both sexual and epistemological, and thereby to arrive at a new philosophy whose mode of expression is ventriloquistic.

Michel Butor's reading of Baudelaire's life, in *Histoire Extraordinaire: Essay on a Dream of Baudelaire's,* suggests that Baudelaire himself might be included among the ventriloquists. While a thorough study of the text of Baudelaire's life lies beyond the scope of this book, it is striking how closely Butor's description of Baudelaire follows Baudelaire's description of Guys. Baudelaire's illness, well documented by himself and others, provides the background for a convalescent narrative written into the text of his life.[40] The illness renders Baudelaire a lifelong convalescent; the assignment of a financial guardian renders him a child. Butor reads this latter loss of responsibility as a loss of manhood: "The imposition of the legal guardianship in 1844 castrated [dévirilisé]

---

40. Baudelaire's notes on his physical condition are included in the *Journaux intimes* and the *Fusées*. His illness, like Nietzsche's, has been mythified by members of both the literary and medical professions. The decadents themselves take up this theme. See, for example, Maurice Barrès, "La folie de Charles Baudelaire," *L'oeuvre de Maurice Barrès*, ed. Philippe Barrès, with a preface by François Mauriac (Paris: Au Club de l'Honnête Homme, 1965), 1:390–401, 432–42. This essay was first published in *Taches d'Encre* (5 November–5 December 1884). Baudelaire is one of Lombroso's favorite degenerates; see *Genio e follia* (Turin: Fratelli Bocca, 1882), as well as *L'uomo di genio* and *Genio e degenerazione* (Palermo: Remo Sandron, 1897). Claude Pichois, in *Baudelaire: Etudes et témoignages* (Neûfchatel: Baconnière, 1967), continues the medicoliterary discussion, citing both Baudelaire's correspondence and five doctoral theses in medicine written in the 1920s on Baudelaire's illness. A more recent and more extensive discussion of Baudelaire's syphilis can be found in Roger L. Williams, *The Horror of Life* (Chicago: University of Chicago Press, 1980).

Baudelaire not physically but morally. His organs are intact, of course, but they are only a sign, and henceforth a deceptive one. He is no longer a man, he is only a child or a woman [il n'est qu'un enfant ou une femme]." This eviration and feminization, according to Butor, influence both his personal relationships and poetic activity so radically that Baudelaire himself assumes the guise of a woman in both spheres: "This does not prevent him from desiring women, from sleeping with them, or at least with one of them, but when he does so he is a woman who desires a woman. Under his man's suit, he is a Lesbian. In *La Fanfarlo,* his alter ego, Samuel Cramer, has published a volume of verse, *Les Orfraies* (*The Ospreys*), under the female pseudonym of Manuela de Monteverde."[41] For Butor, however, this feminization is but a sort of flirtation with transvestitism and merely ("il n'est qu'une femme") prepares the stage for a final *coup de théâtre:*

> Achilles never declares himself more strongly as a virile hero than among the women's clothes he was wearing on Scyros, among the daughters of Lycomedon.
>
> The *mundus muliebris* is thus the necessary theatre of the appearance of genius. The more voluminous the female garments, the more decisive the victory of the poet who tears them to shreds.
>
> Hence we understand why the Lesbian becomes the very symbol of the apprentice poet, of the man who has not yet published. Publication will reveal this superior man hidden under a woman's dress and role [sous une robe et rôle de femme].[42]

This superman in the guise of a woman apparently needs his *robe* and *rôle de femme* only to gestate his ideas; the final and important poetic performance is the triumphant return of virility.[43] Here

---

41. Michel Butor, *Histoire Extraordinaire: Essay on a Dream of Baudelaire's,* trans. Richard Howard (London: Jonathan Cape, 1969), 50; trans. of *Histoire extraordinaire: Essai sur un rêve de Baudelaire* (Paris: Gallimard, 1961).

42. Ibid., 55–56.

43. The effeminate Clark Kent is a paler version of this Achilles who rips off his womanly garments to reveal the superman underneath.

Butor's reading of Baudelaire seems to be a repetition of the narrative of *Le peintre de la vie moderne,* for in the final paragraph of the section "L'artiste, homme du monde, homme des foules, et enfant," Guys's rapid sketching is portrayed as a frenetic duel, a series of feints and lunges:

> Maintenant, à l'heure où les autres dorment, celui-ci est penché sur sa table, dardant sur une feuille de papier le même regard qu'il attachait tout à l'heure sur les choses, s'escrimant avec son crayon, sa plume, son pinceau, faisant jaillir l'eau du verre au plafond, essuyant sa plume sur sa chemise, pressé, violent, actif, comme s'il craignait que les images ne lui échappent, querelleur quoique seul, et se bousculant lui-même. (*Le peintre,* 693)

> [So now, at a time when others are asleep, Monsieur G. is bending over his table, darting on to a sheet of paper the same glance that a moment ago he was directing towards external things, skirmishing with his pencil, his pen, his brush, splashing his glass of water up to the ceiling, wiping his pen on his shirt, in a ferment of violent activity, as though afraid that the image might escape him, cantankerous though alone, elbowing himself on. (Mayne, 12)]

The virile organ is put to the test and the convalescent seems no longer to need his *rôle de femme.* The virility Guys regains is not, however, that to which Andrea Sperelli will return, for Guys's virile organ is a prosthetic one. Butor's suggestion that femininity and supervirility are linked in a superhero fashion is intriguing, but it is not at all clear that prosthetic virility excludes a *rôle de femme.* On the contrary, it would seem that the convalescent's feminization needs to be preserved in order that his *organe viril* not be a literal one. Guys's occupation of the woman's body, if not Baudelaire's, must remain aesthetic, for it is, in a professional sense, his occupation. His goals are achieved principally through his immersion in the feminine, in the *mundus muliebris.*

In the texts of both Nietzsche and Baudelaire, a definition of woman as all surface and no interiority facilitates the convalescent's occupation of her. In a breathtaking sentence, Baudelaire describes "la femme":

> L'être qui est, pour la plupart des hommes, la source des plus vives, et même, disons-le à la honte des voluptés philoso-phiques, des plus durables jouissances; l'être vers qui ou au profit de qui tendent tous leurs efforts; cet être terrible et incom-municable comme Dieu (avec cette différence que l'infini ne se communique pas parce qu'il aveuglerait et écraserait le fini, tandis que l'être dont nous parlons n'est peut-être incompréhen-sible que parce qu'il n'a rien à communiquer); cet être en qui Joseph de Maistre voyait *un bel animal* dont les grâces égayaient et rendaient plus facile le jeu sérieux de la politique; pour qui et par qui se font et défont les fortunes; pour qui, mais surtout *par qui* les artistes et les poètes composent leurs plus délicats bijoux; de qui dérivent les plaisirs les plus énervants et les douleurs les plus fécondantes, la femme, en un mot, n'est pas seulement pour l'artiste en général, et pour M. G. en particulier, la femelle de l'homme. (*Le peintre,* 713)

> [The being who, for the majority of men, is the source of the liveliest and even—be it said to the shame of philosophic pleasures—of the most lasting delights; the being towards whom, or on behalf of whom, all their efforts are directed; that being as terrible and incommunicable as the Deity (with the difference that the Infinite does not communicate because it would thereby blind and overwhelm the finite, whereas the creature of whom we are speaking is perhaps only incompre-hensible because it has nothing to communicate); that being in whom Joseph de Maistre saw a *graceful animal* whose beauty enlivened and made easier the serious game of politics; for whom, and through whom, fortunes are made and unmade; for whom, but above all *through whom,* artists and poets create their most exquisite jewels; the source of the most exhausting pleasures and the most productive pains—Woman, in a word, for the artist in general and Monsieur G. in particular, is far more than just the female of man. (Mayne, 29–30)]

Baudelaire's emphases on *un bel animal* and *par qui* underline the process I have been describing. Though the expulsion of woman in

Le peintre is less dramatic than that in *Il piacere*, it takes place nonetheless as a denial of her existence as a subject or as an agent in the world of art. The contrast between the two uses of *par qui* is striking: fortunes may be made and unmade by the woman as an agent, but works of art are composed by the artist who expresses himself through, by means of, the woman. A denial of consciousness (*un bel animal*) is necessary in order that the woman may become a vehicle, a body emptied of spiritual content. A creature who "perhaps" has nothing to communicate becomes the artist's principal means of communication by lending her attributes to one who, presumably, can render them conscious. His poetic voice, his visual message is transmitted through this body.

In the case of Constantin Guys, immersion in the *mundus muliebris* is crucial for the attainment of his goal, the representation of modernity: "Il s'agit, pour lui, de dégager de la mode ce qu'elle peut contenir de poétique dans l'historique, de tirer l'éternel du transitoire" (*Le peintre,* 694) ["He makes it his business to extract from fashion whatever element it may contain of poetry within history, to distil the eternal from the transitory" (Mayne, 12)]. As a concretization of "le transitoire, le fugitif," fashion plays an important role in Guys's project. Indeed, the absence of the transitory element is figured as an absence of clothing, as a naked woman: "En le supprimant, vous tombez forcément dans le vide d'une beauté abstraite et indéfinissable, comme celle de l'unique femme avant le premier péché" (*Le peintre,* 695) ["By neglecting it, you cannot fail to tumble into the abyss of an abstract and indeterminate beauty, like that of the first woman before the fall of man" (Mayne, 13)]. The *bel animal* is, then, more precisely a clotheshorse, for what better object of "modern" contemplation can there be than a being inseparable from her ever-changing costume?

> Quel poète oserait, dans la peinture du plaisir causé par l'apparition d'une beauté, séparer la femme de son costume? Quel est l'homme qui, dans la rue, au théâtre, au bois, n'a pas joui, de la manière la plus désintéressée, d'une toilette savamment composée, et n'en a pas emporté une image inséparable de la beauté de celle à qui elle appartenait, faisant ainsi des deux, de la femme et de la robe, une totalité indivisible? (*Le peintre,* 714)

[What poet, in sitting down to paint the pleasure caused by the sight of a beautiful woman, would venture to separate her from her costume? Where is the man who, in the street, at the theatre, or in the park, has not in the most disinterested of ways enjoyed a skilfully composed toilette, and has not taken away with him a picture of it which is inseparable from the beauty of her to whom it belonged, making thus of the two things—the woman and her dress—an indivisible unity? (Mayne, 31)]

A *robe* and *rôle de femme* are thus as inseparable from each other as they are inseparable from Guys's project. Rather than, as Butor had described, dramatically ripping off his *vêtements de femme*, Guys the painter (if not Baudelaire the poet) is intent upon adding to his wardrobe:

Tout ce qui orne la femme, tout ce qui sert à illustrer sa beauté, fait partie d'elle-même; et les artistes qui se sont particulièrement appliqués à l'étude de cet être énigmatique raffolent autant de tout le *mundus muliebris* que de la femme elle-même. (*Le peintre,* 714)

Ainsi M. G. s'étant imposé la tâche de chercher et d'expliquer la beauté dans la *modernité,* répresente volontiers des femmes très parées et embellies par toutes les pompes artificielles. (*Le peintre,* 718)

[Everything that adorns woman, everything that serves to show off her beauty, is part of herself; and those artists who have made a particular study of this enigmatic being dote no less on all the details of the *mundus muliebris* than on Woman herself. (Mayne, 30)]

[Having taken upon himself the task of seeking out and expounding the beauty in *modernity,* Monsieur G. is thus particularly given to portraying women who are elaborately dressed and embellished by all the rites of artifice. (Mayne, 34)]

In these passages the body of the woman seems merely a support for
her fashionable finery; it adds an undulating movement that better
displays the sheen of satin. But her body is not only a mannequin for
the display of "le transitoire, le fugitif, le contingent, la moitié de
l'art" (*Le peintre*, 695) ["the ephemeral, the fugitive, the contingent,
the half of art" (Mayne, 13)]; it also, paradoxically, figures "l'autre
moitié . . . l'éternel et l'immuable" ["the other half . . . the eternal
and the immutable"] necessary, according to Baudelaire, to art. The
terms of Baudelaire's argument are overturned by this body, for the
corps should presumably correspond to the contingent element in art,
and the *âme* to the enduring form that the artist distills from that
corps. Yet art that ignores the contingent element is figured as the
body of a woman "avant le premier péché," and in attempting to
describe "La modernité" (section 4), Baudelaire gives the example of
the oldest profession in the world:

> En pareille matière, il serait facile et même légitime de raisoner
> *a priori*. La corrélation perpétuelle de qu'on appelle *l'âme* avec
> ce qu'on appelle *le corps* explique très bien comment tout ce qui
> est matériel ou effluve du spirituel représente et représentera
> toujours le spirituel d'où il dérive. Si un peintre patient et minu-
> tieux, mais d'une imagination médiocre, ayant à peindre une
> courtisane du temps présent, *s'inspire* (c'est le mot consacré)
> d'une courtisane de Titien ou de Raphaël, il est infiniment prob-
> able qu'il fera une oeuvre fausse, ambiguë et obscure. L'étude
> d'un chef-d'oeuvre de ce temps et de ce genre ne lui enseignera
> ni l'attitude, ni le regard, ni la grimace, ni l'aspect vital d'une
> de ces créatures que le dictionnaire de la mode a successivement
> classées sous les titres grossiers ou badins d'*impures,* de *filles en-
> tretenues,* de *lorettes* et de *biches.* (*Le peintre,* 696)

> [In a matter of this kind it would be easy, and indeed legitimate,
> to argue *a priori*. The perpetual correlation between what is
> called the "soul" and what is called the "body" explains quite
> clearly how everything that is "material," or in other words an
> emanation of the "spiritual," mirrors, and will always mirror,
> the spiritual reality from which it derives. If a painstaking,
> scrupulous, but feebly imaginative artist has to paint a courte-
> san of today by Titian or Raphael, it is only too likely that he

will produce a work that is false, ambiguous and obscure. From the study of a masterpiece of that time and type he will learn nothing of the bearing, the glance, the smile or the living "style" of one of those creatures whom the dictionary of fashion has successively classified under the coarse or playful titles of "doxies," "kept women," *lorettes,* or *biches.* (Mayne, 14)]

The example cited threatens to undermine the Platonic terms of Baudelaire's argument; by observing the transitory element, *le corps,* we may arrive at the eternal element, *l'âme,* yet what is eternal about the most recent practitioners of the oldest profession in the world is precisely a function of the body. As though perceiving this menace, Baudelaire hastens to add that courtesans are by no means a privileged object ("Le lecteur comprend d'avance que je pourrais vérifier facilement mes assertions sur de nombreux objets autres que la femme" ["I need hardly tell you that I could easily support my assertions with reference to many objects other than women"); yet the two examples that follow receive no further attention in *Le peintre.* Ships are nowhere to be found, and horses, when they do appear, are merely accessories to a larger scene. Nor do these examples possess in such a marked degree the qualities necessary to Baudelaire's argument—an "immutable" form and function dressed in the style of its age. The courtesan thus offers herself as a ready-made work of art.

But there is yet another sense in which Constantin Guys does not abandon his *robe* and *rôle de femme* and in which he appears not as a superman but as a ventriloquist. The woman of "L'éloge du maquillage" (section 11) is, like Guys, an expert in the art of painting; her canvas is her body, her goal to use artifice to improve upon nature:

Ainsi, si je suis bien compris, la peinture du visage ne doit pas être employée dans le but vulgaire, inavouable, d'imiter la belle nature et de rivaliser avec la jeunesse. . . . Qui oserait assigner à l'art la fonction stérile d'imiter la nature? (*Le peintre,* 717)

[Thus, if you will understand me aright, face-painting should not be used with the vulgar, unavowable object of imitating fair Nature and of entering into competition with youth. . . .

Who would dare to assign to art the sterile function of imitating Nature? (Mayne, 34)]

An artist in her own right, the cosmetician serves as a model for Constantin Guys in two senses; her painting prescribes an aesthetic at the same time as she and her painting pose for his contemplation. But if the woman is already a work of art, has already improved upon nature, then what aesthetic governs Guys's representation of her? To which of the age-old camps—mimesis or *cosmesis*—does Guys belong? Does he improve upon artifice as the woman improves upon nature, or is he guided by an aesthetic of imitation which Baudelaire holds in contempt? The text provides no answer, but it would seem that Guys imitates artifice: "Les artistes qui se sont particulièrement appliqués à l'étude de cet être énigmatique raffolent autant de tout le *mundus muliebris* que de la femme elle-même" (*Le peintre,* 714) ["Those artists who have made a particular study of this enigmatic being dote no less on all the details of the *mundus muliebris* than on Woman herself" (Mayne, 30)]. While both Butor and Baudelaire seem to understand *mundus muliebris* as "the woman's world," glossing it with the French *monde,* the expression may also refer, as it does in the Book of Esther, to the woman's cosmetics.[44] It is, then, the woman's art of painting which inspires Guys, in which he must immerse himself and through which (*par qui*), finally, his message is transmitted. If "la peinture du visage" is the model for his aesthetic, then Guys's paintings of "les femmes et les filles" speak through those painted faces and ornamented

---

44. Baudelaire explicitly glosses the French *monde* as *mundus*: "Enfin, je veux dire que le goût précoce du monde féminin, *mundi muliebris*, de tout cet appareil ondoyant, scintillant et parfumé, fait des génies supérieurs" ["Un mangeur d'opium"] (1:499). ["In short, I mean that the precocious taste for the feminine world, *mundus muliebris*, for all that undulating, glittering and perfumed paraphernalia, fashions superior genius."] The French *monde* does not retain the double meaning of the Latin *mundus*, which (like the related Greek *kosmos*) means both "world" and "ointments, adornments." The biblical *mundus muliebris*, instead refers quite specifically to ointments in the phrase "et accipiant mundum muliebrem, et caetera ad usus necessaria." Liber Esther, 2:3, *Biblia sacra iuxta vulgatam clementinam* (Madrid: Biblioteca de Autores Cristianos, 1977). The Douay Rheims translation renders *mundus muliebris* as "ornaments"; the Revised Standard Version reads, "let their ointments be given them" (Book of Esther 2:3).

bodies, through nature improved by artifice. His poetic "voice" is projected through that woman's body, which supposedly had nothing to communicate. Here, with the aid of the convalescent-artist, that body begins to speak and turns out to have everything to communicate. The woman is a work of art, but a mute one: "C'est une espèce d'idole, stupide peut-être" ["She is a sort of idol, perhaps a stupid one"], a sort of dummy awaiting animation and occupation by the convalescent. The convalescent's feminization and the artist's androgyny are thus the preparation for, and legitimation of, an act of ventriloquism.

In the preface to the second edition of *The Gay Science*, it is Nietzsche himself who poses as convalescent. His pose is, of course, not unique to this preface; in *Ecce Homo*, Nietzsche presents himself as a lifelong convalescent, "Der Genesende" is one of Zarathustra's incarnations, and the opposition between health and sickness furnishes rhetorical scaffolding in almost all his works.[45] I speak, therefore, of the 1886 preface as a moment in Nietzsche's writings which depends upon and recalls other moments, not as a synecdoche for the *opera omnia* but as the most powerful mise-en-scène of the scene of convalescence.

The convalescent of this preface is strikingly Baudelairean: the steps we have taken slowly, in analyzing and describing the convalescences of Guys and Sperelli, Nietzsche takes in leaps and bounds. The first of these—the expulsion of woman—does not, strictly speaking, occur in these few pages. But if we read the preface against the background of Nietzsche's other writings, against the background of Nietzsche's repeated venomous stabs at "abortive females" and "hysterical bluestockings," at women young and old, we can say the the expulsion of woman is a precondition of Nietzsche's discourse.[46] The accompanying step,

45. One of the most interesting discussions of the rhetoric of sickness in Nietzsche is Pierre Klossowski, *Nietzsche et le cercle vicieux* (Paris: Mercure de France, 1969). The "Lombrosian" response to Nietzsche's rhetoric of sickness and biographical illness is analyzed by Sander Gilman in his article on Nietzsche as "pathogen": "The Nietzsche Murder Case," *New Literary History* 14.2 (1983): 359–72, now in *Difference and Pathology* (Ithaca: Cornell University Press, 1985).

46. Many have written on the function and significance of "woman" in Nietzsche's writings. See, for example, Eric Blondel, "Nietzsche: Life as Metaphor," in *The New Nietzsche: Contemporary Styles of Interpretation*, ed. David B. Allison (New

the liquidation of the crowd, is a similar precondition, which is merely alluded to as the "radical retreat into solitude as a self-defense against a contempt for men,"[47] from which the convalescent slowly emerges. These steps taken, the narrative moves rapidly to the feminization of the convalescent and his ventriloquizing speech.

The convalescences of Constantin Guys and of Andrea Sperelli were the scene of artistic creation; Nietzsche's convalescence is the scene and source of philosophic creation. Convalescence is the preface to the work; it is placed, mimetically, before its product: "Gratitude pours forth continually, as if the unexpected had just happened—the gratitude of a convalescent—for *convalescence* [Genesung] was unexpected. 'Gay Science': that signifies the Saturnalia of a spirit who has patiently resisted a terrible, long pressure—patiently, severely, coldly, without submitting but also without hope—and who is now all at once attacked by hope, the hope for health, and the *intoxication* of convalescence" (*GS,* 32). As in the texts of Baudelaire and D'Annunzio, convalescence is linked to intoxication as well as to rebirth and childhood: "One returns *newborn* . . . with merrier senses, with a second dangerous innocence in joy, more childlike" (*GS,* 37). And once again, the convalescent occupies a space in-between, an interstice. *The Gay Science,* Nietzsche tells us, contains April weather. As a month of passage between seasons, April is most appropriate to the convalescent's passage between health and sickness. Interestingly enough, April and September are described in *Il piacere* as "i mesi neutri" ["the neuter months"]; Sperelli's preference is for the month in which his own convalescence takes place: "Il settembre. E più feminino" (*Il piacere,* 178) ["September. It is more feminine"]. Nietzsche, however, changes the terms of the expected analogy, for in his text April marks not a passage from the winter behind (or sickness) to

York: Dell, 1977); Jacques Derrida, *Spurs: Nietzsche's Styles/Eperons: Les styles de Nietzsche,* trans. Barbara Harlow (Chicago: University of Chicago Press, 1979); Sarah Kofman, *Nietzsche et la scène philosophique* (Paris: Union Générale d'Editions, 1979); and Luce Irigaray, *Amante marine: De Friedrich Nietzsche* (Paris: Minuit, 1980).

47. Friedrich Nietzsche, *The Gay Science,* ed. and trans. Walter Kaufmann (1887; New York: Vintage Books, 1974), 33, hereafter cited in the text, abbreviated *GS.*

the summer ahead (or health) but a moment between different sicknesses, between one winter and another: "One is instantly reminded no less of the proximity of winter than of the triumph over the winter that is coming, must come, and perhaps has already come" (GS, 32). Thus, though the convalescent experiences a "hope for health," the term *summer*, which might fulfill that hope and represent such a stable state, is absent. It is not health that is desirable but the perpetuation of convalescence. A stable state of health would represent precisely that which Nietzsche attacks, the immobilization of perspective and consequent scleroticization of values:

> You see that I do not want to take leave ungratefully from that time of severe sickness whose profits I have not yet exhausted even today. I am very conscious of the advantages that my fickle health gives me over all robust squares [Vierschrötigen des Geistes]. A philosopher who has traversed many kinds of health and keeps traversing them, has passed through an equal number of philosophies; he simply *cannot* keep from transposing his states every time into the most spiritual form and distance: this art of transfiguration *is* philosophy. (GS, 35)

The convalescent-philosopher moves along the vector between "kinds of health"; like Nietzsche's skater, dancer, and tightrope walker, he never touches stable ground, never stops at either pole, never adopts a rigidly fixed perspective. Philosophy occupies this space in-between, the space of convalescence.

It is by traversing kinds of health that Nietzsche comes to see all previous philosophy as "a misunderstanding of the body" and, as Eric Blondel puts it, as the equivalent of a hysterical symptom, of the body's conversion into language.[48] The valorization of convalescence is thus an important epistemological move. The thematization of the body and its symptoms aims to establish a new, nonhysterical relationship between the body and thought. Rather than being tyrannized by the ways in which "the sick body and its

---

48. "As a sickness of culture, man is born in and by bad conscience which, itself, ushers in this meta-phorical, quasi *hysterical*, and displaced language: it is the body's symptomatic *conversion* into language" (Blondel, 151).

needs unconsciously urge, push and lure the spirit" (GS, 34), the convalescent-philosopher would lend an ear to these urgings. Yet in order to hear and give voice to these whisperings, the convalescent must, paradoxically, occupy the hysterical body par excellence: the woman's body. Giving voice is figured as giving birth: the convalescent-philosopher is an incarnation of what Nietzsche calls the "mother-type": "We philosophers are not free to divide body from soul as the people do; we are even less free to divide soul from spirit. We are not thinking frogs, nor objectifying and registering mechanisms with their innards removed: constantly we have to give birth to our thoughts out of our pain and, like mothers [mütterlich], endow them with all we have of blood, heart, fire, pleasure, passion, agony, conscience, fate and catastrophe" (GS, 35–36). That the figuration of the philosopher as mother is linked to the scene of convalescence is confirmed by passages in both The Gay Science and The Genealogy of Morals, where Nietzsche makes explicit yet another stage in the convalescent's feminization. The convalescent's otium turns out to be a lying-in, for one of the sicknesses from which he recovers is that of the bad conscience: "The bad conscience is an illness, there is no doubt about that, but an illness as pregnancy is an illness."[49] True, this sort of pregnancy does not always receive a positive prognosis, but in the case of the artist and philosopher such pregnancy is the matrix of a new art and philosophy, as in these two passages from The Gay Science:

Pregnancy has made women kinder, more patient, more timid, more pleased to submit; and just so does spiritual pregnancy produce the character of the contemplative type, which is closely related to the feminine character: it consists of male mothers. (GS, 129)

Consider a continually creative person, a "mother" type in the grand sense, one who knows and hears nothing any more

49. Friedrich Nietzsche, The Genealogy of Morals, trans. Walter Kaufmann and R. J. Hollingdale (New York: Vintage Books, 1969), 88. The genealogy of Nietzsche's discourse on pregnancy can, of course, be traced to Plato's Symposium, where it is Diotima (in yet another act of ventriloquism) who expounds upon the pregnancy of the soul.

except about the pregnancies and deliveries of his spirit.
(*GS*, 326)

The philosopher's spiritual activity is described in terms of and inscribed in the body of the woman, the very body that is an object of vituperation and horror in Nietzsche's writings. Once again, woman is expelled so that her attributes might be parcelled out; her mothering function is appropriated by the philosopher as a figure for an altered relationship between the body and thought. "Woman" is a particularly seductive ground for this metaphorical operation: vituperation of women frequently relies upon a rhetorical move whereby manifestations of woman's body are said to be "all in the mind," while the activity of her mental faculties is said to be controlled by her body. The mother is thus chosen to represent the new philosopher not only because of her creative fecundity but also because of this supposed, peculiarly female, interanimation between mind and body.

The "children" born of the convalescent-philosopher's pregnancy are his truths, not *the* truth but a number of truths born of his mobile perspective. In relation to traditional notions of truth as an essence to be sought behind appearance, these truths must appear to be untruths, little more than personal whimsy. Woman, as all surface and no interiority, thus comes to represent *both* the alluring deceptiveness of the notion of truth as essence *and* the new philosopher's truths.[50] So it is that at the end of the 1886 preface, the philosopher ventriloquizes:

50. I refer the reader to Derrida's discussion of "truth" and "woman" in *Spurs*: "There is no truth of woman but it is because that abyssal divergence of truth, this non-truth is 'truth.' Woman is a name of this non-truth of truth." Derrida, *Spurs/Eperons*, 51 (translation modified). Derrida both critiques and continues the Nietzschean critique of the hermeneutic model. The polemical thrust of Nietzsche's style seems to become Derrida's polemical thrust, as Derrida himself enacts a double expulsion of woman from the text. That is to say, Derrida continues to identify feminism with the castrating woman and appears to reserve for "himself" the (non)position of the "third woman." In the present context, this would seem to be yet another occupation that facilitates ventriloquism. See also his remarks in James Creech, Peggy Kamuf, and Jane Todd, "Deconstruction in America: An Interview with Jacques Derrida," *Critical Exchange* 17 (Winter 1985): 28–32.

We no longer believe that truth remains truth when the veils are withdrawn; we have lived too much to believe this. Today we consider it a matter of decency not to wish to see everything naked, or to be present at everything, or to understand and "know" everything.

"Is it true that God is present everywhere?" a little girl asked her mother; "I think that's indecent"—a hint for philosophers! One should have more respect for the bashfulness with which nature has hidden behind riddles and iridescent uncertainties. Perhaps truth is a woman who has reasons for not letting us see her reasons? Perhaps her name is—to speak Greek—*Baubo?* (*GS,* 38)

The convalescent-philosopher's truth is spoken through the woman's body: Baubo, the personification of the female genitals, is the site of knowledge. It is this act of ventriloquism which Blondel seems to have in mind when he characterizes "Nietzsche's 'ontology' as feminine, or even as gynecological, for this ontology speaks of being as a woman who has no being."[51] Blondel's phrase "as a woman" can, it seems to me, be read as bearing both a metaphorical and a metonymic sense: woman is metaphor of being and the gender adopted by the philosopher when he speaks of being.

Andrea Sperelli's ventriloquist moment, like Nietzsche's, is situated at the end of the narrative of convalescence. But unlike Nietzsche and Constantin Guys, Sperelli is not "toujours, spirituellement, à l'état du convalescent"; in books 3 and 4, Sperelli will return to a *vita del Piacere,* to that life of flirtations and seductions which had ended, temporarily, in the "mortale ferita" that had necessitated his convalescence. After the curtains close upon the scene of convalescence, he will once again feel "come un malato che abbia perduto ogni fiducia di guarire. . . . Gli pareva che di nuovo l'antica lebbra gli si dilatasse per l'anima" (*Il piacere,* 258) ["like a sick man who has lost all faith of getting well. . . . It seemed to him that the old leprosy once again was spreading through his soul"]. The concluding section of book 2, then, represents the culmination of Sperelli's convalescence and of his unstable

51. Blondel, 156.

conversion to the ivory tower of art. It is here that we find the diary of a *turris eburnea* and androgyne, Maria Ferres.

Maria Ferres's diary has been described as the weakest point in the novel, as a discordant note in the stylistic register of *Il piacere,* as an anachronistic and artificial use of a technique of the eighteenth-century novel.[52] However we might choose to evaluate it, Maria's diary intrudes on the convalescent narrative and its omniscient narrator, marking a moment of rupture in the text. This moment of rupture is, I propose, due less to the diary form than to the identity of its fictional author. As I have noted, the narrative of book 2 is interspersed with sonnets and bits of poetry offered as the fruits of Sperelli's disquisitions on aesthetics. Such a combination of poetry and aesthetic theory already constitutes a disturbance of the form of the novel (if, that is, the novel is held to contain a minimum of metalanguage). Yet that disturbance appears motivated by the novel since it is, after all, Sperelli who rediscovers his poetic voice, Sperelli who elaborates a theory of aesthetics, Sperelli who projects a "poema moderno," "una lirica veramenta moderna," "un grande studio di decadenza" (*Il piacere,* 160) ["a modern poem," "a truly modern lyric," "a great study of decadence"]. Guided by this narrative logic, the reader-critic might reasonably expect Sperelli's works to appear as the culmination of his convalescence. The inclusion of Maria Ferres's diary thus appears unmotivated, the caprice of a young novelist. But there is something more disquieting about the diary than possible lack of skill on the part of the author. The diary clears a particular space for a voice that, as we have observed, receives special descriptive attention: "Era una voce ambigua, direi quasi bisessuale, duplice, androginica; di due tim-

---

52. Eurialo De Michelis's judgment is typical: "The defect becomes worse when, outside of the protagonist's representation, it is a matter of staging, in the form of an autonomous character, the 'spirituality,' 'ideality,' 'the intimate life of the heart,' all the 'things of the soul' in whose name the moral judgment is given. We allude to the attempted portrait of the exquisitely internal charms of Maria Ferres (accompanied by the usual charms, more accessible to touch). These charms are not content to be merely asserted but aspire to dictate introspective pages of a diary attributed to her, a facile expedient already typical of love novels. As introspection, these and other such pages that precede and follow the diary are among the weakest in the book." De Michelis, *Tutto D'Annunzio* (Milan: Feltrinelli, 1960), 80.

bri" (*Il piacere,* 169) ["It was an ambiguous voice, I would almost say bisexual, double, androgynous, of two timbres"]. Maria thus has interesting potential, both as a ventriloquist and for a ventriloquist, potential Sperelli cannot resist exploiting in book 4.

"Il timbro feminile appunto ricordava *l'altra*" (*Il piacere,* 170) ["The feminine timbre recalled the other woman"]: the feminine timbre which so reminds Andrea of Elena Muti supplies the foundation for the climactic episode of book 4. Outside the scene of convalescence, the ex-convalescent does not attempt to project his own voice through the woman but rather the voice of another woman. Sperelli is not as unabashed as Des Esseintes, but his game is the same; rather than simply handing Maria a dialogue to memorize, he coaxes her into following his script. Maria remains unaware of the part she plays in this "staged scene":[53]

—Quanto mi piace!
Andrea tremò. Non era quello lo stesso accento di Elena nella sua sera della dedizione? Non erano le stesse parole? Egli le guardave la bocca.
—Ripeti.
—Che cosa?
—Quello che hai detto.
—Perché?
—E una parola tanto dolce, quando tu la pronunzii... Tu non puoi intendere... Ripeti.
Ella sorrideva, inconsapevole, un po' turbata dallo sguardo singolare dell'amante; quasi timida.
—Ebbene... mi piace!
—Ed io?
—Come?
—Ed io... a te...?
Ella, perplessa, guardava l'amante che le si torceva ai piedi, convulso, nell'aspettazione della parola ch'egli voleva strapparle.
—Ed io?

53. For a discussion of this episode as a "staged scene," see Paolo Valesio, "Genealogy of a Staged Scene: *Orlando furioso,* V," *Yale Italian Studies* n.s. 1 (Spring 1980): 5–31.

—Ah! Tu... mi piaci.

—Così, così... Ripeti. Ancòra!

Ella consentiva, inconsapevole. Egli provava uno spasimo ed una voluttà indefinibili. (344)

["How I love it!"

Andrea trembled. Was that not the very accent Elena had used the evening she had given herself to him? Were those not the same words? He looked at her mouth.

"Say that again."

"What?"

"What you said."

"Why?"

"It is such a sweet word, when you say it... You cannot understand... Say it again."

She smiled, unaware, a bit disturbed by her lover's odd expression, almost shy.

"Well then, I love it!"

"And me?"

"What?"

"And me? Do you love me?"

Perplexed, she looked at her lover writhing at her feet, convulsed, as he waited for the word that he wanted to draw from her.

"And me?"

"Oh! I love you."

"Yes, like that. Say it again!" She consented, unsuspecting.

He experienced an indefinable voluptuous spasm.]

Maria thus unknowingly repeats the words Elena had pronounced on the occasion of her first tryst with Andrea. Elena's voice and Elena's words issuing from Maria's body send Sperelli into an erotic fury, much as Flaubert's dialogue issuing from the ventriloquist had excited Des Esseintes. His "cupo ardore" is checked only by a tragic slip of the tongue when, in the climactic episode, he calls out Elena's name in the most inappropriate of circumstances:

Nel letto, smarrita, sbigottita, innanzi al cupo ardore del forsennato, ella gridava:

— Ma che hai? Ma che hai?

Ella voleva guardarlo negli occhi, conoscere quella follia; ed egli nascondeva il viso, perdutamente, nel seno, nel collo, ne' capelli di lei, ne' guanciali.

A un tratto, ella gli si svincolò dalle braccia, con una terribile espressione d'orrore in tutte quante le membra, più bianca de' guanciali, sfigurata più che s'ella fosse allora allora balzata di tra le braccia della Morte.

Quel nome! Quel nome! Ella aveva udito quel nome! (*Il piacere*, 363)

[In bed, before the dark ardor of the crazed man, bewildered and frightened, she cried, "What's wrong with you? What's the matter?" She wanted to look into his eyes, to know that madness. And he buried his face, passionately, in her breast, her neck, her hair, in the pillows.

Suddenly she disentangled herself from his arms with a terrible expression of horror in all of her limbs, whiter than the pillows, her face more distorted than if she had just then leapt from the arms of Death.

That name! That name! She had heard that name!]

This slip of the tongue is, of course, tragic for Andrea only insofar as Maria is unwilling to continue with the script. The voice of Elena issuing from the body of Maria is not merely a substitute for Elena but an exquisitely tantalizing object of desire in itself. Only Maria-with-the-voice-of-Elena can satisfy Sperelli's penchant for combining the "sacred" with the "profane." Thus, at the end of the novel Sperelli has fully exploited the "timbro feminile" of Maria's voice by transforming her into an unknowing and unwilling ventriloquist; Elena's tone becomes dominant when Maria assumes Elena's position in *amor profano*.

What becomes of "il timbro maschile, basso e un poco velato" (*Il piacere*, 169) ["the masculine timbre, low and slightly veiled"]? It is this voice, I suggest, which recounts the story of the *amor sacro* between Andrea and Maria. The record of her stay at Schifanoia, Maria's diary is also the account of her gradual surrender to Andrea's charms. What at first seemed a change of focus in the narrative turns out to be a sharpening of focus on Sperelli, for the count's opinions, tastes, and professions of love are so faithfully recorded that the diary is, for the most part, a repetition of the narrative that precedes it. Maria, the ivory tower, begins to lean when she admits to deriving pleasure from this repetition. "Tutte queste particolarità le ho dal disegnatore; provo uno strano piacere a ricordarle, a scriverle," reads one entry, and another: "Se ci fosse un mezzo, potrei riprodurre ogni modulazione della sua voce" (*Il piacere,* 201, 214) ["I have all of these details from the artist; I feel a strange pleasure in remembering them, in writing them down." "If there were a means, I could reproduce every modulation of his voice"]. What is added is corroboration of the emotions already expressed by Andrea; when Maria notes that "la sua voce è come l'eco dell'anima mia" (*Il piacere,* 269) ["his voice is like the echo of my soul"], it is because *her* voice is, in fact, the echo of his. Her diary is the fulfillment of Sperelli's goal:

> Egli voleva possedere non il corpo ma l'anima, di quella donna; e possedere l'anima intera, con tutte le tenerezze, con tutte le gioie, con tutti i timori, con tutte le angosce, con tutti i sogni, con tutta quanta insomma la vita dell' anima; e poter dire: — Io sono la vita della sua vita. (*Il piacere,* 180)

> [He wanted to possess not the body but the soul of that woman, to possess her entire soul, with all its tenderness, all its joys, all its fears and anguish and dreams, with all the life of the soul and be able to say: —I am the life of her life.]

These are exactly the terms in which the narrator presents Maria Ferres's diary:

> Maria Ferres era rimasta sempre fedele all'abitudine giovenile di notar cotidianamente in un suo Giornale intimo i pensieri, le gioie, le tristezze, i sogni, le agitazioni, le aspirazioni, i rimpianti, le speranze, tutte le vicende della sua vita interiore, componendo quasi un Itinerario dell'Anima. (*Il piacere,* 193)

> [Maria Ferres had always remained faithful to the habit of her youth of noting daily in her personal diary the thoughts, joys, sadnesses, dreams, anxieties, aspirations, regrets, hopes, all

the events of her inner life, composing an Itinerary of the Soul.]

The diary, then, bears witness to Maria's possession by Andrea, a possession that, as the phrase suggests, verges on the demonic. Possession is characterized as the repetition of the same words, sentiments, and desires that Andrea had used and expressed; the more Maria's voice resembles Andrea's, the more complete his possession of her. His occupation of her is total when she makes it possible for him to say, "Io sono la vita della sua vita":

—Quando, sul limite del bosco, egli colse questo fiore e me l'offerse, non lo chiamai *Vita della mia vita?*

Quando ripassammo pel viale delle fontane, d'innanzi a quella fontana, dove egli prima aveva parlato, non lo chiamai *Vita della mia vita?*

Quando tolse la ghirlanda dall'Erma e la rese a mia figlia, non mi fece intendere che la Donna inalzata ne' versi era già decaduta, e che io sola, io sola ero la sua speranza? Ed io non lo chiamai *Vita della mia vita?* (*Il piacere*, 209)

[When, at the edge of the woods, he picked this flower and offered it to me, did I not call him *Life of my life?*

When we returned by the fountain path, in front of that fountain where he had first spoken, did I not call him *Life of my life?*

When he took the garland from the bust and gave it to my daughter, did he not give me to understand that the Woman glorified in verse had already fallen, and that I alone was his hope? And did I not call him *Life of my life?*]

Andrea thus succeeds in ventriloquizing; if the feminine timbre is Elena's, the masculine timbre is Andrea's. Seen against the background of the convalescences of Guys and Nietzsche, Sperelli's erotic success is a measure of his artistic failure; the masculine ideas he succeeds in transmuting into the woman's body are concupiscient rather than aesthetic. In fact, he communicates his "disease" to Maria: "Una cosa oscura e bruciante è in fondo a me, una cosa ch'è apparsa d'improvviso come un'infezione di morbo e che incomincia a contaminarmi il sangue e l'anima, contro ogni volontà, contro ogni rimedio: il Desiderio" (*Il piacere,* 215–16) ["There is something dark and burning within me, something that has appeared suddenly like an infection and has begun to contaminate my blood and soul, against all will, against all cure: Desire"]. Maria Ferres's diary thus appears to be soundly motivated precisely as testimony to Sperelli's failure as an artist, his failure to discover a new relationship between the body and thought. Sperelli's ventriloquism, like Des Esseintes's, is limited to the degradation of his muse. His convalescence ended, Sperelli writes no more but returns to "l'antica lebbra"; the unstable convert to "l'Arte . . . l'Amante fedele" now turns to Maria, "l'Amante Ideale."

Sperelli's artistic failure could seem a parody of Guys's and Nietzsche's "successes," a reliteralization of the man's occupation of the woman, only if *Il piacere* is considered apart from D'Annunzio's other novels. Sickness and convalescence are major preoccupations in his prose works, both before and after *Il piacere,* and in the 1921 *Notturno* convalescence appears once again as the scene of artistic creation. The narrator of *Notturno* succeeds where Sperelli had failed. Here sickness and convalescence truly become an alibi for a new prose style, a style that D'Annunzian criticism prefers to that of the earlier novels precisely because of its "modernity."[54] But the convalescent of *Notturno* is successful in another sense as well, for he achieves this stylistic modernity by adopting a "feminine" mode of writing.

D'Annunzio assumes the guise of D'Annunzio in *Notturno;* the narrator lies in the dark, convalescing from a wound to the eye like that D'Annunzio had actually received in World War I. This temporary blindness ("Ho gli occhi bendati") represents a material obstacle to the writer's practical functioning, and a new mode of writing must be devised for him:

M'era vietato il discorrere e in ispecie il discorrere scolpito;

---

54. One of the commonplaces of D'Annunzian criticism, this preference is so widespread as to deserve a separate article in which to list all of its proponents. Ermanno Circeo's intelligent overview of D'Annunzian criticism describes the major camps: *Il D'Annunzio "notturno" e la critica dannunziana di un settantennio* (Pescara: Trimestre, 1975).

né m'era possibile vincere l'antica ripugnanza alla dittatura e il pudore segreto dell'arte che non vuole intermediarii o testimonii fra la materia e colui che la tratta. L'esperienza mi dissuadeva dal tentare a occhi chiusi la pagina. La difficoltà non è nella prima riga ma nella seconda e nelle seguenti. Allora mi venne nella memoria la maniera delle Sibille che scrivevano la sentenza breve su le foglie disperse al vento dal fato.[55]

[All forms of discourse, and in particular sculpted discourse, were forbidden me. Nor could I overcome my old revulsion against dictation and the secret modesty of art that wants no intermediaries or witnesses between the matter and him who forms it. Experience dissuaded me from attempting the page with eyes closed. The difficulty lies not in the first line, but in the second and all those that follow. Then I remembered the technique of the Sibyls, who wrote their short sentences on sheets of paper dispersed to the winds by Fate.]

Strips of paper are cut for the convalescent in order that he might adopt the sibylline mode of writing, which is the technical motivation of the prose style, impressionistic and lapidary, of *Notturno*. The ventriloquism of *Notturno* is less corporeal than that of *Le peintre de la vie moderne*, *The Gay Science*, or *Il piacere*, but not thereby less complete. The image of the blindfolded narrator becomes, in *Il compagno dagli occhi senza cigli*, the image of his muse: "La malattia e la morte son le due muse bendate che ci conducono in silenzio a scoprire la spiritualità delle forme" ["Sickness and death are the two blindfolded muses who lead us in silence to discover the spirituality of forms"].[56] If Sperelli degraded his muse and mislaid his poetic inspiration, the convalescent-narrator of *Notturno* is at once inspired writer and his own muse. Far from parodying and

55. Gabriele D'Annunzio, *Notturno*, in *Prose di ricerca di lotta, di comando, di conquista, di tormento, d'indovinamento, di rinnovamento, di celebrazione, di rivendicazione, di liberazione, di favole, di giochi, di baleni, Tutte le opere di Gabriele D'Annunzio*, ed. Egidio Bianchetti (Milan: Mondadori, 1954), 1:172.

56. D'Annunzio, *Il compagno dagli occhi senza cigli*, in *Prose di ricerca* (Milan: Mondadori, 1956), 2:614.

then abandoning the decadent ideologeme of convalescence, D'Annunzio brings it to perfection in *Notturno*. The twist given the
scene of convalescence in *Il piacere* is thus a comment upon Sperelli's
exaggerated opinion of his own talents, rather than a lack of talent
on the part of D'Annunzio; it is a deviation from the Baudelairean
rhetoric of convalescence which relies upon that rhetoric for its
interpretation.

[3]   *The Shadow of Lombroso*

Class Bodies

The scene of convalescence is not exclusively Baudelairean territory, nor is the Baudelairean rhetoric of sickness the only, or even the dominant, rhetoric of sickness in D'Annunzio's early prose works. Convalescents appear in *Terra vergine, Le novelle della Pescara,* and *L'Innocente,* but theirs are "Lombrosian" convalescences. In the Baudelairean rhetoric, lingering sickness is the ground for artistic creation that cannot be reduced to a mere symptom; the "sick" subject is a reader of his own "symptoms" and reads them as signs. The Lombrosian model, instead, interprets mental and spiritual activity as little more than physiological tics; the "sick" subject produces symptoms but is unable to read them as anything at all. Both rhetorics posit particular relationships between the body and thought, but their symptomatologies and conclusions are so divergent that it would perhaps be more precise to speak of "bodies" rather than "the body." In D'Annunzio's early prose works, different social classes and sexes are presented as so many different bodies, as sites of different relationships of the body to thought. Only the upper-class male appears as a Baudelairean convalescent, while the Lombrosian convalescents are female and/or lower class. These Lombrosian convalescences are the scene not of conversion to artistic creation and ventriloquism but of hysterical conversion, the threshold of dementia, mystic delirium (as Nordau would say), and an introduction to, rather than a taking leave of, perversion. Their case studies thus constitute countertexts to the convalescences of Andrea Sperelli and the narrator of *Notturno*.

The very adoption of a rhetoric of sickness, be it Baudelairean or Lombrosian, is a thematization and valorization of the corporeal, which may be construed in various ways. A description of physiological illness may be a mode of presentation of psychic imbalance, an inroad to the unconscious; it may be the most effective strategy for drawing attention to the body per se; it may represent the dark side of a celebration of sexuality. D'Annunzio exploits all three of these possibilities in his novelistic attempts to describe relationships between bodies and thought, between sexuality and psychology. D'Annunzian critics, it seems, deem these questions unworthy of literary and philosophical exploration. Judging from their reactions to the thematization of sexuality in D'Annunzio's works (merged in their minds with lascivious anecdotes concerning their author), one wonders if they also hid Dr. Freud's writings from their daughters.[1]

D'Annunzio's adoption of the Lombrosian and Baudelairean rhetorics of sickness is part of his search for a language with which to describe and explain psychological formations, which he describes in the preface to *Trionfo della morte:*

> Uscendo dalle figure, dico che la lingua italiana non ha nulla da invidiare e nulla da chiedere in prestito ad alcun'altra lingua europea non pur nella rappresentazione di tutto il

---

1. Lest this judgment seem too malicious, I quote P. Giuseppe Venturini, who, in a 1980 issue of *Quaderni del Vittoriale,* quotes from one of his earlier articles, a "faithful echo," as he puts it, of the polemic against D'Annunzio: "Since he wrote under the domination of vanity and lust, which suffocate all true inspiration, his entire opus is neither art nor poetry but merely an 'enormous bamboozling' ['enorme corbellatura']. Thus condemned to a monotonous and oppressive repetition, his is an illusory fecundity. D'Annunzio's heroes, male and female, all have the same flesh, his flesh rotten with lust: false creatures just as their author is false. . . . In their verbose falsity, their maniacal hyperboles and obsessive repetitions, their boundless nullity of useless and sick beings, his heroes are a portrait of D'Annunzio himself, the 'superlative histrion.' This is why D'Annunzian characters of whatever sex, age, and condition all have the same voice, the voice of their author refractory to every idea and every ideal." P. Giuseppe Venturini, "Spiritualità e religiosità di D'Annunzio," *Quaderni del Vittoriale* 4 (July–August 1980): 43.

moderno mondo esteriore ma in quella degli "stati d'animo" più complicati e più rari in cui analista si sia mai compiaciuto da che la scienza della psiche umana è in onore.

E gli psicologi appunto, poichè sembra che i nuovi romanzieri d'Italia inclinano a questa scienza, gli psicologi in ispecie hanno per esporre le loro introversioni un vocabolario d'una ricchezza incomparabile, atto a fermare in una pagina con precisione grafica le più tenui fuggevoli onde del sentimento, del pensiero e fin dell'incoercibile sogno.[2]

[Leaving figures aside, I assert that the Italian language has nothing to envy and nothing to borrow from any other European language, not even in the representation of the modern external world nor yet in that of the most complicated and unusual "states of mind" that any analyst has ever congratulated himself on since the inauguration of the science of the human psyche.

And it is precisely the psychologists (since the new Italian novelists tend toward this science) who have a vocabulary of an incomparable richness with which to present their introversions, a vocabulary capable of capturing on the page with graphic precision the most tenuous and fleeting waves of feeling, thought, and even irrepressible dream.]

My project, in this chapter, is to take seriously the extensive D'Annunzian project, which touches upon and distinguishes between different classes and sexes. The distinction that results from the copresence of Baudelairean and Lombrosian rhetorics is not, however, between upper and lower classes, male and female protagonists as, respectively, mind and body. The coupling of a Lombrosian rhetoric with women and the lower classes is not simply the result of a denial of the body by the upper classes and its consequent displacement onto the "other." The two rhetorics of sickness cannot be neatly labeled "Baudelairean upper-class male" and "Lombrosian lower-class female," for while the Baudelairean rhetoric of convalescence seems not to be employed in the service of female characters,

---

2. Gabriele D'Annunzio, *Trionfo della morte*, in *Prose di romanzi, Tutte le opere di Gabriele D'Annunzio*, ed. Egidio Bianchetti (Milan: Mondadori, 1955), 1:655.

the Lombrosian rhetoric is extended to all the classes and sexes studied by Lombroso himself. The peasants of *Terra vergine* and *Le novelle della Pescara,* the virgins Orsola and Anna of *Le novelle della Pescara,* Tullio Hermil of *L'Innocente* can all be included under the Lombrosian label. The last character—upper-class male—does indeed belong to a special category, for it is the Lombrosian etiology of genius which characterizes him or, rather, with which he, as narrator, characterizes himself. What is at stake in these D'Annunzian texts is the invention of several different bodies and physiopsychologies, as we shall see.

The problem of "class bodies" has occupied both Jean-Paul Sartre and Michel Foucault, whose hypotheses may help clarify D'Annunzio's position not because either explains D'Annunzio's texts but because neither is adequate to do so. In relation to the ideology of D'Annunzio's novels and novellas, Sartre's hypothesis regarding the bourgeoisie's denial of the body appears to be ancient history. In the *Critique of Dialectical Reason,* Sartre analyzes the suppression of the body, its denial and constraint through dress, as an essential part of the bourgeoisie's constitution of itself as a class. The body, according to Sartre, stands as "the presence in the oppressor of the oppressed in person," and is thus negated and enslaved just as the proletariat is oppressed and enslaved by the bourgeoisie:

> Lastly, more directly and more profoundly, the act of social oppression is itself repeated here together with all its significations: he is really oppressing the workers when he subjects the universality of his own body to countless constraints; it is the worker as the universal class that he destroys within himself or conceals under *artificially* produced particularities; and it is the repression of the workers' revolt against hunger, cold, fatigue, etc., which he exercises here against fatigue, cold and hunger as revolts *of his body.*[3]

D'Annunzio's texts do not, of course, sing the praises of hunger and fatigue, but they do explore and magnify different bodies,

3. Jean-Paul Sartre, *Critique of Dialectical Reason,* trans. A. Sheridan Smith (London: New Left Books, 1976), 772; trans. of *Critique de la raison dialectique,* vol. 1 (Paris: Gallimard, 1960).

celebrate and mourn them. It is as though the denial of the universality of the body has been so effective as to give rise to entirely different bodies belonging to different classes. Were Sartre's hypothesis directly complementary to D'Annunzio's texts, one would expect the combination of the Lombrosian rhetoric with an upper-class protagonist to be avoided at all costs, for it is the Lombrosian rhetoric that characterizes, for example, the swarming peasant mob of *Trionfo della morte,* as well as the bestial peasants of *Terra vergine.* But instead, the assiduously avoided combination is that of the Baudelairean rhetoric applied to female and lower-class characters. Those characters appear to be "all body" because of the type of consciousness attributed them, rather than because the body has been expelled *tout court* from the experience of the upper-class male protagonist.

Foucault, in *The History of Sexuality,* presents a thesis that is the inverse of Sartre's and equally problematic. Arguing against the *doxa* according to which sexuality has only recently emerged from the depths of repression, Foucault locates the body and sexuality on the other side of the barricades: "There is little question that one of the primordial forms of class consciousness is the affirmation of the body; at least, this was the case for the bourgeoisie during the eighteenth century. It converted the blue blood of the nobles into a sound organism and a healthy sexuality. One understands why it took such a long time and was so unwilling to acknowledge that other classes had a body and a sex—precisely those classes it was exploiting."[4] According to Foucault, it was necessary to deny that laboring classes had a body in order to instrumentalize that body and, at the same time, to distinguish social classes by producing sexuality as a distinctive feature that the lower classes lacked. Sexuality as discourse becomes the property of the upper classes, that which the lower classes have not, rather than a common bond between classes. Still, as with Sartre's thesis, Foucault's hypothesis is only partly pertinent to D'Annunzio's texts, where we find both upper- and lower-class bodies, both upper- and lower-class sexualities. The lower-class body participates not in sexuality as

4. Michel Foucault, *The History of Sexuality,* trans. Robert Hurley (New York: Vintage Books, 1980), 1:126; trans. of *L'histoire de la sexualité* (Paris: Gallimard, 1976).

discourse but in a sort of mute bestiality that seems little more than an instinctive urge to copulate. Eros in the lower-class body retains no relative autonomy from other bodily functions. The upper-class body, on the other hand, participates in a sexuality that is nothing other than an amalgamation of "perversions," of turnings from the path of that urge. The upper classes have a physiological psychology; the lower, a physiology. Woman occupies an intermediary position in this schema, for she shares in both bestiality and sexuality; her psychology is continually threatened by her physiology.

Flora and Fauna of the Virgin Terrain

The atavism of *Terra vergine* approaches the extremes of Lombroso's evolutionary delirium and zoological scenarios. Indeed, it is difficult to claim that the physiologies and physiognomies that populate this virgin terrain, unviolated by consciousness, are aberrant. They are socially and physically atavistic, and behavior occurs naturally, that is to say, in the absence of thought. The otherness of the lower-class body is marked not by contrast to an upper-class character (for none appear in *Terra vergine*), but by similitude to animals: the characters of *Terra vergine,* without exception analogized to animals, are arguably not even "human."[5] Such an attribution of bestiality to human beings appears to be almost a personification of animals, an elevation rather than a degradation. Only the characters' names would seem to mark them as human actors, yet in two cases—"Dalfino" and "la gatta"—their already folkloristic names are those of animals, and in a third story three characters are grouped under the title "Bestiame."[6] Lust (*lascivia, lussuria,* not

5. For a more extensive discussion of bestial analogies in *Terra vergine* and of D'Annunzio's "Darwinism" in relation to that of Giovanni Verga, see Pietro Gibellini, "*Terra vergine* e il verismo dannunziano," *Logos e mythos: Studi su Gabriele D'Annunzio* (Florence: Olschki, 1985), 155–81.

6. The 1882 "Bestiame" appears to be a rewriting of Verga's 1880 "La lupa," a rewriting rather than "theft," for the sex of the protagonists has been changed. In "La lupa," a mother-in-law seduces her son-in-law; in "Bestiame," it is a father-in-law who seduces his daughter-in-law. Such a change of sex may alter the ideology thus embodied. For a discussion of a similar change of sex (between

eros) is the dominant motive, lust that leads to sickness or death or is itself a kind of sickness and death.

The most animalesque of these creatures become part of the landscape in satisfying their lust. In the title story, Tulespre is barely distinguishable from the pigs he tends; his desire parallels theirs: "E andavano alle querci della Fara, i porci a saziarsi di ghiande, Tulespre a fare all'amore" ["And they went to the Fara oaks, the pigs to eat their fill of acorns, and Tulespre to make love"].[7] The "acorn" that will satisfy Tulespre is Fiora, who, always surrounded by the goats she herds, "rassomigliava una pantera" (*Terra vergine,* 6) ["resembled a panther"]. The names Tulespre and Fiora simply label a natural osmosis, as desire grows, plantlike, over the landscape and through the human actors:

A poco a poco in quel refrigerio l'arsura gli svampava dai pori; dai mucchi di fieno intorno vaporante gli saliva su per le narici calde una voluttà di profumo; in fondo all'erba udiva brulichii d'insetti; provava su la pelle, ne' capelli vellicamenti di corpuscoli strani; e il cuore gli palpitava al ritmo selvaggio dello stornello di Fiora. (*Terra vergine,* 4)

[Little by little, the burning heat escaped from his pores in that cool spot. From the moldering haystacks a voluptuous aroma rose to his hot nostrils; at the roots of the grass he heard the swarming of insects. On his skin and in his hair he felt ticklings of strange corpuscles, and his heart palpitated to the savage rhythm of Fiora's stornello.]

Oedipus Rex and Anna of *La città morta*) see Paolo Valesio, "Il coro degli Agrigentini," *Quaderni del Vittoriale* 36 (1982): 65–92. A more striking example of the substitution of one relative for another, and the difference it makes, may be found in Freud and Breuer's *Studies on Hysteria* in the case of "Katharina." The 1895 Freud changed Katharina's tale such that the father who seduced her becomes, in Freud's text, an uncle. Sigmund Freud and Josef Breuer, *Studies on Hysteria,* vol. 2 of *The Standard Edition of the Complete Psychological Works of Sigmund Freud,* trans. James Strachey (London: Hogarth Press and the Institute of Psychoanalysis, 1956), 134, hereafter cited in the text.

7. Gabriele D'Annunzio, *Terra vergine,* in *Prose di romanzi, Tutte le opere,* ed. Egidio Bianchetti (Verona: Mondadori, 1968), 1:3.

No intellect intervenes to select or reject these thoughts of nature; no more consciousness can be attributed to the human actors than to the goat that witnesses their copulation: "Una testa nera di capra sbucò tra il fogliame guardando con le miti iridi gialle quel groppo vivo di membra umane" (*Terra vergine,* 7) ["The black head of a goat poked out among the leaves and, with gentle yellow irises, watched that living tangle of human members"]. Their lusty story is repeated by Dalfino ("pareva proprio un delfino" [8] ["she looked just like a dolphin"]), and Zarra ("Ma che superba fiera era quella Zarra!" [9] ["What a proud beast was that Zarra!"]) in the story "Dalfino," where jealousy and murder conclude their idyll ("Gli si fece addosso come una tigre" [12] ["He attacked him like a tiger"]); by Nara ("china, con la schiena al solleone, colla gonna bianca, pareva una pecora" [13] ["bent over, with her back to the burning sun and her white skirt, she looked like a sheep"]), and Malamore in "Fiore fiurelle"; by Biasce and Zolfina in "Campane"; by Tora and Mingo in "La gatta"; by father and daughter-in-law in "Bestiame"; by Ziza, Iori, and Mila in "Ecloga fluviale." In "Ecloga fluviale," sensual burgeoning is presented as healthy despite its final expression as jealous rage and murder:

> Ora fioriva così Mila, come una pianta, come un tronco tutto felice di germini.... La vita per quel corpo di femmina si effondeva con un fluore vittorioso di umori sani; e da quella sanità emergeva un senso vergine e lucido delle cose, naturalmente. Tutta la pompa delle forze muliebri aveva già trionfato nell'essere; ora Mila in quella pompa si adagiava con la serenità semplice di chi non pensa, di chi non teme, di chi non sa. (*Terra vergine,* 56)

> [Now Mila blossomed, like a plant or a trunk adorned with buds. . . . Life spread through that female body with a victorious flux of healthy humors. And from that health there emerged, naturally, a virgin and lucid sense of things. All the pomp of womanly forces had already triumphed in her being. Now Mila settled into that pomp with the simple serenity of one who does not think, does not fear, does not know.]

An archaic physiology of humors is adopted to describe desire in a human plant. The relationship of body to thought, in these peasant bodies, is reduced to a relationship between the body and behavior governed by instincts.

Despite his reptilian name, Fra' Lucerta appears the least animalesque of these personified plants and animals and the most similar to the characters of *Le novelle della Pescara*. Unlike the mute Toto and the idiot Cincinnato, Fra' Lucerta is capable of speech and is even literate. Unlike Rocco's typhoid fever or Zolfina's smallpox, Fra' Lucerta's disease is desire itself. A rhetoric of sickness is linked once again to the tension between "conversion" and "perversion." Fra' Lucerta's vocation impedes the flow of the "umori sani" of "Ecloga fluviale"; his attempts to turn from the path of his lust sicken him and qualify his lust as a sort of primitive sexuality rather than as the bestiality that motivates the other characters of *Terra vergine*. His are not, however, the consciousness-sharpening fevers of Andrea Sperelli's convalescence, but the obfuscating ones of desire:

> Una febbre lenta gli bruciava il sangue e gli sconvolgeva l'intelletto. La carne ed il sangue martoriati per tanti anni ora insorgevano terribili ed imperiosi come due schiavi inferociti ad affermare il loro diritto. (*Terra vergine*, 40)

> [A slow fever burned his blood and troubled his intellect. His flesh and blood, martyred for so many years, now rose up to assert their rights, imperious and terrible like two enraged slaves.]

Enslaved flesh revolts against an ineffectual intellect, recalling Sartre's description of the body as "the presence in the oppressor of the oppressed in person." Yet here D'Annunzio takes the part of the "oppressed," of the body; his demystifying move reduces Fra' Lucerta's faith to a displacement of his lust (or, in Nietzschean terms, a misunderstanding of the body). Both Fra' Lucerta's spiritual vocation and his desire for Mena are named by the same term: "La fede era per lui una febbre, gli dava la vertigine e l'allucinazione" (*Terra vergine*, 39) ["Faith was a fever for him, it gave him vertigo and hallucinations"]. The two seemingly antagonistic fevers are one, his lust is his faith: "Quando il sangue e la carne gli si ribellavano sotto la tonaca, si gettava lì davanti a quel suo Cristo nero contorcendosi come una serpe rotta nella schiena" *(Terra vergine,* 39) ["When his flesh and blood rebelled beneath his frock, he threw himself down before his black Christ, writhing like a serpent with a broken back"]. Fra' Lucerta's devotion is but a symptom of his physiological condition.

Of the stories of *Terra vergine,* only "Fra' Lucerta" can be said to pose the question of the relationship of physiology to thought; elsewhere there is only behavior. The concerns of this story, its "Christian" theme and the demystifying framework in which it is set, are taken up again in *Le novelle della Pescara.*

The Novellas of Pescara and Vienna

In *Le novelle della Pescara,* the interaction between body and thought, sexuality and psychology in the lower-class woman's body is more complex than it is in the peasant body of *Terra vergine.* Like *Terra vergine,* these tales are archaizing; the hagiographic titles of the first two stories suggest that the edifying lives of two saintly virgins, "La vergine Orsola" ["The Virgin Ursula"] and "La vergine Anna" ["The Virgin Anna"] are about to be recounted. The narratives that gloss those titles, however, undermine rather than satisfy expectation. As the name of the mother of the Virgin Mary suggests, "La vergine Anna" does indeed end in beatification, but it is, it seems, epilepsy and imbecility, rather than mystical illumination and miracle working, which are so rewarded. "La vergine Orsola" is the story of a brutal rape, an even more brutal abortion, and a squalid death. The irony of this latter title is underscored by the choice of "Orsola" as the name of the "vergine sverginata." In fact, in the earlier version of the same tale which appeared in *Il libro delle vergini,* the protagonist's name was Giuliana (who becomes, instead, a bourgeois convalescent in *L'Innocente*). "Juliana," the name of a minor saint, is, in *Le novelle della Pescara,* replaced by "Ursula" who, of course, had a more illustrious career as leader

of the legendary eleven thousand virgins.[8] The choice of such a
notoriously saintly virgin for a tale of rape leaves little doubt as to
the story's demystificatory aims. Both stories associate Christianity
with illness, idiocy, and ignorance; a "naturalistic" mode is adopted
not to give an accurate, scientific description of peasant society but
to degrade and critique an ideology. Like Nietzsche in the *Antichrist*, D'Annunzio employs a rhetoric of sickness in order to critique
Christianity.

"La vergine Orsola" is, in fact, a convalescent narrative. In the
opening section of the story, Orsola, dying from typhoid fever,
offers a blackened tongue to receive the host and falls into a
stupor as extreme unction is administered her. Her rebirth as a
convalescent is thus all the more unexpected and dramatic. Here,
as in *Il piacere*, convalescence is characterized as both rebirth, "una
seconda nascita," (*Le novelle*, 79) and as a state of forgetfulness: "Il
passato si dileguava, si assopiva in fondo alla memoria, non risor-
geva più" (*Le novelle*, 91) ["The past faded away and slumbered in
a far corner of her memory; it surfaced no more"]. But the combination of convalescence and the lower-class female body is the site of
a different chemistry; the description of Orsola's convalescence
emphasizes not the acuity of consciousness but the cellular activity
of her body:

> La convalescenza era lunga e lenta, ma già un senso mite di
> sollievo cominciava a spargersi per le membra, a liberare il
> capo. Per quella sana nutrizione di albume e di carne muscolare
> un sangue novello si produceva: i polmoni dilatati ora larga-
> mente dall'aria vivificavano il sangue carico di sostanze; e i

---

8. D'Annunzio does seem to have incorporated elements of Saint Juliana's
life into his tale of the "vergine Orsola." According to *The Saints: A Concise
Biographical Dictionary*, ed. John Coulson (New York: Hawthorn Books, 1958),
"Juliana was the child of noble, wealthy Florentine parents, and on the death of
her father was educated under the direction of St. Alexis Falconieri, her uncle.
Refusing to marry, she entered the Servite Third Order and was instrumental
in founding its conventual branch, of which she became superior. She showed
great devotion to the eucharist. On the day of her death being unable to take
food she was deprived of communion, and a host was placed at her request on
her breast; it miraculously penetrated into her body, enabling her, says tradition,
to be nourished with the sacrament of Christ's body."

tessuti irrigati dall'onda tiepida e rapida si colorivano ricomponendosi, si rinnovellavano nelle piaghe di decubito, si ricoprivano di cute a poco a poco; e le attività cerebrali a quell'affluire operavano sicure; e le innervazioni negli organi sensorii non più perturbate rendevano limpida la sensazione; e sul cranio i bulbi capilliferi rigermogliavano densi; e da quel riordinamento delle leggi meccaniche della vita, da quel dispiegarsi di energie prima latenti che la malattia aveva provocate, da quella intensa brama che la convalescente aveva di vivere e di sentirsi vivere, da tutto, lentamente, quasi in una seconda nascita, una creatura migliore sorgeva. (*Le novelle,* 79)

[Her convalescence was long and slow, but already a mild sense of relief began to spread through her members and free her head. A new blood was formed from that healthy diet of albumen and meat: the lungs, now amply dilated by the air, vivified the blood rich in substance; and her tissues, irrigated by that tepid and swift wave of blood, took on new color and recomposed themselves, were renewed in bedsores and were re-covered with cutis little by little. And cerebral activites functioned securely with that influx, the innervations of the sensory organs, no longer disturbed, rendered sensation limpid. On the cranium the capilliferous bulbs resprouted densely. And from that reordering of the mechanical laws of life, from that unfolding of energies previously latent which the sickness had caused, from that intense lust for life and for feeling alive which the convalescent had, from everything, a better creature slowly arose, as if in a second birth.]

The woman's physiology interacts differently with her psychology; while Sperelli experienced convalescence as the death of desire, Orsola experiences it as the discovery of desire. Once again convalescence introduces a new relationship between the body and thought, but it is hunger and lust that are awakened in the lower-class female body:

L'istinto della fame si ridestava vivissimo, come più chiara si faceva la conscienza. Quando dal forno di Flaiano saliva nell'aria l'odore caldo del pane, Orsola chiedeva; chiedeva con un accento di mendicante famelica, tendeva la mano, supplicando alla sorella. Divorava rapidamente, con un godimento brutale di tutto l'essere, guardando d'intorno se qualcuno tentasse strapparle di tra le mani il cibo, in sospetto. (*Le novelle,* 79)

[The instinct of hunger reawakened with vigor as her consciousness became ever clearer. When the warm aroma of bread rose from Flaiano's bakery, Orsola asked for it, asked in the tone of a famished beggar. She held out her hand, begging her sister. She devoured it rapidly, with a brutal enjoyment in all her being, looking about her suspiciously to make sure that no one would try to snatch the food away from her.]

Orsola, who had spent her short life transmitting "la piccola dottrina, i piccoli canti della religione" (*Le novelle,* 80) ["the little doctrine, the little songs of religion"] to the children of the village, now turns away from and forgets her faith. Her convalescence is the scene not of her conversion to art but of her introduction to perversion. The vision that appears on the tabula rasa of this convalescent's mind is not that of "l'Arte ... l'Amante fedele," but of the brothel that faces her bedroom window. The observation of the brothel's commerce becomes her pastime and works a sort of anticonversion in the virgin convalescent: "Così, nella vergine, si accendeva la brama. Il bisogno dell'amore, prima latente, si levava ora da tutto il suo essere, diventava una tortura, un supplizio incessante e feroce da cui ella non sapeva difendersi" (*Le novelle,* 90) ["The need for love, previously latent, now rose from all her being, became a torment, an incessant and ferocious torture against which she knew not how to defend herself"]. The awakening of lust in Orsola suggests a retrospective reading of her former devotion to charitable works as a defense mechanism rather than as successful sublimation. The virgin who never once touched a child's curls or kissed a childish brow now undertakes a correspondence with a soldier, her future violator acting as go-between. Thus the forgetfulness of convalescence allows her sexuality to develop, bloom, erupt. As Freud might have said, a repression has been lifted.

Indeed, D'Annunzio's life of a virgin calls to mind what might be called the novellas of Vienna: the 1895 Freud-Breuer *Studies on*

Hysteria. A dialogue between Pescara and Vienna can be created by emphasizing the narrative structure of Freud's clinical studies and the clinical gaze of D'Annunzio's narrative. Just as D'Annunzio's account of Orsola's life begins in medias res with a description of her illness and near death, so do Freud and Breuer begin their portraits of hysterical patients (women all, virgins most) with descriptions of their symptoms, their paralyses, coughs, and tics. In D'Annunzio's text, a long convalescence follows that illness; in Freud and Breuer's text, the doctors' treatment follows the opening symptomatology. That treatment mimes the structure of convalescence: the patient must forget everything in order to remember all. Memory plays a major role in both the scene of convalescence and in hysteria, for Freud and Breuer diagnosed hysteria as an illness deriving from memory: "Hysterics suffer mainly from reminiscences" (Freud-Breuer, 7). The cure, then, consists in forcing—through hypnosis, through pressure upon the forehead or eyes—the patient to remember. But while the patient's task is to remember and tell all, the doctor's task is, notably in the case of Frau Emmy von N., to induce forgetfulness, to induce the traits of convalescence. Freud in this case study does little more than "wipe away" memories of which Frau von N. has no shortage. Indeed, the magic eraser of hypnosis presents such dizzying possibilities that Freud gets carried away, and toys with Frau von N.'s memory to such an extent that Dr. Breuer must rebuke him.[9] Yet Freud's joke well represents the crudeness and cruelty of this early technique, for the successful cure is, it seems, a state of partial amnesia:

I saw Frau von N. again in the spring of the following year

9. "In this connection I ventured upon a practical joke in one of my suggestions to her. This was the only abuse of hypnosis—and a fairly innocent one at that—of which I have to plead guilty with this patient. I assured her that her stay in the sanatorium at '*-tal*' ('-vale') would become so remote to her that she would not be able to recall its name and that whenever she wanted to refer to it she would hesitate between '*-berg*' ('-hill'), '*-tal*,' '*-wald*' ('-wood') and so on. This duly happened and presently the only remaining sign of her speech-inhibition was her uncertainty over this name. Eventually, following a remark by Dr. Breuer, I relieved her of this compulsive paramnesia" (Freud-Breuer, 79–80).

at her estate near D———. She had grown stout, and looked in flourishing health. She had felt relatively well during the nine months that had passed since the end of her last treatment. . . . It was during these days, too, that she made her complaints about gaps in her memory, "especially about the most important events" . . . from which I concluded that the work that I had done two years previously had been thoroughly effective and lasting. (Freud-Breuer, 83–84)

Lombroso, who was familiar with Charcot's work and mentions Freud and "Breus" in *Genio e degenerazione,* was more blunt in recognizing the power relationship that structures the hypnotic situation:

Quello che più importa a noi è la facilità a subire la così detta suggestione ipnotica, con cui l'ipnotizzatore sostituisce alla volontà del paziente la propria.... E', l'isterico ipnotizzato, insomma, un automa obbediente, senza spontaneità, alla volontà altrui.[10]

[What is most important to us is the facility to submit to so-called hypnotic suggestion, with which the hypnotizer substitutes the patient's will with his own. . . . In short, the

10. Cesare Lombroso and G. Ferrero, *La donna deliquente, la prostituta e la donna normale* (Turin: L. Roux, 1893), 610. Lombroso's understanding of Freud and Breuer's work was, however, less than complete: "Nell'isteria però, come Janet e Binet in Francia, Breus [*sic*] e Freud a Vienna dimostrarono, si tratta essenzialmente d'una lesione intellettiva, dipendente piuttosto dagli scambi delicati corticali che da alterazioni cerebrali grossolane" ["In hysteria, however, as Janet and Binet in France, Breus [*sic*] and Freud in Vienna have demonstrated, it is essentially a question of an intellective lesion, dependent upon fine cortical exchanges rather than upon crude cerebral alterations"]. Lombroso, *Genio e degenerazione* (Palermo: Remo Sandron, 1897), 23. The power relationship that structures hypnotic treatment, and psychoanalytic treatment in general, has been the subject of much recent feminist criticism. A most useful bibliography can be found in *Diacritics* (Spring 1983), an issue titled "A Fine Romance: Freud and Dora."

hypnotized hysteric is an automaton obedient to the will of
others, with no spontaneity.]

Freud's playfulness with Frau Emmy von N.'s memory, his displea-
sure with disobedient patients such as Dora, his repeated complaints of "dissatisfaction" when Miss Lucy R. fails to produce the
information desired indicate that Freud is not far from subscribing
to Lombroso's assessment. At the time of the *Studies on Hysteria,* of
course, Freud was still in dialogue with the alienists, still arguing
against theories of *dégénérescence.* In the penultimate paragraph of
Emmy's case, Freud dismisses the degeneration theory and in so
doing also demonstrates that he has not yet become "Freud," does
not yet know what will truly differentiate his theory from those of
his predecessors: "To describe such a woman as a 'degenerate' would
be to distort the meaning of that word out of all recognition. We
should do well to distinguish between the concepts of 'disposition'
and 'degeneracy' as applied to people; otherwise we shall find
ourselves forced to admit that humanity owes a large proportion of
its great achievements to the efforts of 'degenerates'" (Freud-
Breuer, 104). The argument is certainly a weak one for, we have
seen, Lombroso does indeed attribute humanity's conquests to the
efforts of degenerates. Freud has not yet elaborated the theory of
the unconscious which will set him apart from his predecessors,
though the *Studies on Hysteria* set him in the "right" direction. It
is here that Freud begins to read and translate what he calls the
"pictographic script" of the hysteric's body: "We (Breuer and I) had
often compared the symptomatology of hysteria with a pictographic
script which has become intelligible after the discovery of a few
bilingual inscriptions. In that alphabet being sick means disgust"
(Freud-Breuer, 129). This reading/translation is one in which the
key, the Rosetta stone, is held only by Freud. The amnesiac patient,
instead, continues to produce "hieroglyphs," continues, as Frau
Emmy von N. did, to produce symptoms that she herself is incapable of reading and translating: "The therapeutic success on the
whole was considerable; but it was not a lasting one. The patient's
tendency to fall ill in a similar way under the impact of fresh
traumas was not got rid of" (Freud-Breuer, 101). The jumble of
traumatic events that had made her ill continues to convert itself

into tongue clacking and stuttering while the doctor-narrator goes on to become ever more eloquent, ever more skilled as translator.

Similarly, the author of the *Le novelle della Pescara* is not yet "D'Annunzio." By this I do not mean that he is instead a plagiaristic mixture of Maupassant, Flaubert, and Giovanni Verga but that he will work through the Lombrosian rhetoric of sickness employed in these tales in order to arrive at the lyrical antinovels of his maturity. These two contemporaries—the not-yet Freud and the not-yet D'Annunzio—work along parallel tracks, which lead backward toward Lombrosian premises and forward toward non-Lombrosian conclusions. The narrators of "La vergine Anna" and "La vergine Orsola" do not, of course, enter their stories as "Dr. D'Annunzio," but the narrative structures and the problems they pose are similar to those of Freud's case studies. Just as Freud induces the effects of convalescence in order to lift repressions, so does D'Annunzio set up convalescence as the scene of the discovery of desire in "La vergine Orsola." Though not a convalescent narrative, "La vergine Anna" mimes yet other aspects of Frau Emmy von N.'s case study.

Frau von N.'s life was an accumulation of traumas: siblings who threw dead animals at her, brothers who grabbed her on their deathbeds, carriages very nearly struck by lightning, a husband who dropped dead before her very eyes. Anna's biography is similarly, and no less believably, constructed as a series of traumas, beginning with her introduction to life. Her birth is so difficult that Anna is baptized *in utero*. Then, when she is five, the child's clothes catch fire as her mother holds her up to kiss the local patron saint. The trauma leaves her dumb:

> Per le ustioni Anna stette inferma lungo tempo in pericolo. Ella giaceva nel letto, con l'esile faccia esangue, senza parlare, come fosse diventata muta; e aveva negli occhi aperti e fissi un'espressione di stupore immemore più che di dolore. (*Le novelle,* 120)

> [From the burns, Anna lay ill and in danger for a long time. She lay on her bed, her face thin and bloodless, without speaking, as though she had become mute. And in her open

and staring eyes, there was an expression of forgetful stupor
more than of pain.]

It is this "stupore immemore" that will characterize Anna's life;
she is a sort of born amnesiac whose memory manifests itself only
as illness. The narrative follows a sequence of traumas, eclipsing
those moments of Anna's life in which no traumatic event leaves
its impression upon her. Eight years pass, in which "nothing"
happens until Anna's mother dies, trampled to death in church by
the overzealous faithful. Her memory of the event appears in the
form of epilepsy: "Anna, quando vide la madre distesa sul letto
tutta violacea nella faccia e macchiata di sangue, cadde a terra senza
conoscenza. Poi, per molti mesi, fu tormentata dal mal caduco"
(Le novelle, 123) ["When she saw her mother stretched on the bed,
her face all purple and stained with blood, Anna fell to the ground
unconscious. Afterwards, for many months she was tormented by
epilepsy"]. This is not Dostoevskian or even Lombrosian epilepsy,
for Anna receives no genial illumination as a result of her attacks.[11]
Instead, they seem to render her more feebleminded. Four years
later comes another trauma: her father abandons her, leaving her
in the care of relatives who employ her as a sort of serving maid:
"Ella non osava lamentarsi, poiché mangiava il pane nella casa degli
altri. Ma quel supplizio di tutte le ore la rendeva ebete: una
imbecillità grave le opprimeva a poco a poco l'intelligenza indebol-
ita" (Le novelle, 123–24) ["She dared not complain, for she ate her
bread in the house of others. But that continuous torture made
her half-witted: a heavy imbecility little by little oppressed her
weakened intelligence"]. There follows a brief idyll between Anna
and a donkey entrusted to her care, then another trauma: the ass
dies and Anna's epilepsy returns, accompanied by renewed religious
fervor: "Nel 1845 il mal caduco riapparve con violenza; sparve dopo
alcuni mesi. La fede religiosa in quell'epoca divenne in lei più
profonda e più calda" (Le novelle, 127) ["In 1845, her epilepsy
returned with violence; it disappeared after several months. In that
period her religious faith became deeper and more fervent"]. As

11. An avid reader of Dostoevsky, Lombroso similarly associated epileptic
seizures and genial illumination in his studies on genius, L'uomo di genio and
Genio e degenerazione.

D'Annunzio well knew, the association of epilepsy with religious experience is ancient; indeed, in *Trionfo della morte,* Ippolita's epilepsy is described as "il male sacro" ["the sacred disease"], a locution D'Annunzio does *not* use in the tale of the virgin Anna. Epilepsy here is not a sign that marks the chosen; Anna's religious faith appears instead to be a symptom of her epilepsy. It is in this sense that one of the rhetorics of this novella can be seen as Lombrosian; Anna's mystical experiences are portrayed as symptoms of her body, as the side effects of illness.

The demystifying effect of the Lombrosian rhetoric is in contrast to the hagiographic tone that asserts itself as the narrative continues. The connection between illness and faith becomes more complex after the second idyllic interlude in Anna's life, in which she is given a tortoise, which will accompany her thereafter, and considers marrying Zacchiele. Zacchiele, however, loses Anna's already uncertain affection by kicking the tortoise and soon after dies in a flood. This apparent misfortune is in fact providential, for Anna's potential saintliness is reinforced by the preservation of her virginity. At this point, the hagiographic tone becomes dominant.

Her virginity intact, other illnesses begin to manifest themselves in her body. The pulmonary infection that follows Zacchiele's death is Anna's mode of mourning and reinforces her faith. Then, after a brief stay with her paralytic uncle, whose young wife manages to pilfer Anna's belongings, the virgin is received into a convent. By now an elderly woman, Anna begins to exhibit new symptoms:

> Con l'andar del tempo, le estasi si fecero più frequenti. La vergine canuta era colpita a quando a quando da suoni angelici, da echi lontani d'organo, da romori e voci non percettibili agli orecchi altrui. Figure luminose le si presentavano dinanzi, nel buio; odori paradisiaci la rapivano.
>
> Così pel monastero una specie di sacro orrore cominciò a diffondersi, come per la presenza di un qualche potere occulto, come per l'imminenza di un qualche avvenimento soprannaturale. Per cautela, la nuova conversa fu dispensata da ogni obbligo d'opere servili. Tutte le attitudini di lei, tutte le parole, tutti gli sguardi furono osservati, comentati con superstizione. E la leggenda della santità incominciò a fiorire.

Su le calende di febbraio dell'anno di Nostro Signore 1873, la voce della vergine divenne singolarmente rauca e profonda. Poi la virtù della parola d'un tratto scomparve. (*Le novelle*, 155)

[With the passing of time, her ecstasies became more frequent. The white-haired virgin was stricken from time to time with angelic sounds, distant echoes of organs, sounds and voices not perceptible to other ears. Luminous figures showed themselves to her in the darkness; heavenly smells enraptured her.

Thus a sort of sacred horror began to spread throughout the monastery, as if through the presence of some occult power, or through the imminence of some supernatural event. As a precaution, the new lay sister was released from all obligation to perform servile tasks. All of her attitudes, all of her words and glances were observed and commented upon with superstition. And the legend of her sanctity began to blossom.

On February 1 in the year of Our Lord 1873, the virgin's voice became singularly hoarse and deep. Then her power of speech suddenly disappeared.]

In these three paragraphs the hagiographic tone is unmarred by the sort of demystifying insinuations I have noted. The nuns and inhabitants of the village do, in fact, interpret Anna's loss of voice, her olfactory and aural hallucinations as signs of saintliness. The tension between the villagers' interpretation and a potentially demystificatory one creates an ambiguity in the narrator's stance. The hagiographic tone continues until Anna's voice returns and "la fama del miracolo si sparse dal monastero in tutto il paese di Ortona" (*Le novelle*, 157) ["fame of the miracle spread from the monastery throughout the village of Ortona"]. At this point, however, the narrator refers to Anna as "l'inferma" ["the sick woman"], rather than as "la vergine":

Nell'agosto del 1876 sopravvennero nuovi prodigi. L'inferma, quando si avvicinava il vespro, cadeva in uno stato di estasi con catalessia; donde sorgeva poi quasi con impeto. E in piedi, conservando sempre la medesima attitudine, cominciava a parlare, da prima lentamente e quindi gradatamente accelerando, come sotto l'urgenza di un'ispirazione mistica. Il suo eloquio non era se non un miscuglio tumultuario di parole, di frasi, di interi periodi già innanzi appresi, che ora nella sua inconsapevolezza si riproducevano, frammentandosi o combinandosi senza legge. Le native forme dialettali s'innestavano alle forme auliche, s'insinuavano nelle iperboli del linguaggio biblico; e mostruosi congiungimenti di sillabe, inauditi accordi di suoni avvenivano nel disordine. Ma il profondo tremito della voce, ma i cangiamenti repentini dell'inflessione, l'alterno ascendere e discendere del tono, la spiritualità della figura estatica, il mistero dell'ora, tutto concorreva a soggiogare gli animi delle astanti. (*Le novelle*, 157)

[In August of 1876, new prodigies occurred. When the time for vespers neared, the sick woman would fall into state of cataleptic ecstasy, and then rise again almost with violence. Standing, and maintaining always the same position, she would begin to speak, first slowly and then gradually accelerating as if under the urgency of a mystical inspiration. Her eloquence was nothing other than a tumultuous mixture of words, phrases, entire sentences she had learned before and which now, in her unconsciousness, reproduced themselves, fragmented themselves to combine together without law. Forms of her native dialect grafted themselves onto aulic forms and insinuated themselves into the hyperboles of biblical language. Monstrous conjunctions of syllables and unheard-of chords were produced in the disorder. But the deep tremble in her voice, the sudden changes of inflection, the alternating rise and fall of tone, the spirituality of the ecstatic figure, the mystery of the hour, all contributed to subjugating the minds of the onlookers.]

The writing of hagiography gives way to an interpretation of symptoms; the tumult of words which issues from Anna's mouth is not a message from God but the surfacing of her past. Like Frau Emmy von N., whose traumas converted themselves into tongue clacking, Anna's traumas resurface as a sort of idiotic glossolalia.

In the subsequent paragraph, in which her attacks are described in greater detail, the narrator's only epithet for Anna is "l'inferma." Then, having lost her teeth, her hair, and her sense of cleanliness, she forgets even the existence of her beloved tortoise.

At this point, the two interpretations seem to part ways; the characters of the story read Anna's gradual disintegration as a sign from above, while the narrator seems to hold the Lombrosian (and early Freudian) Rosetta stone:

> Ma le suore consideravano la imbecillità e la infermità della donna come una di quelle supreme prove di martirio a cui il Signore chiama gli eletti per santificarli e glorificarli poi nel Paradiso; e circondavano di venerazione e di cure l'idiota. Nell'estate del 1881 apparvero i segni della morte prossima. Consunto e piagato, quel miserabile corpo omai nulla più conservava di umano. Lente deformazioni avevano viziata la positura delle membra; tumori grossi come pomi sporgevano sotto un fianco, su una spalla, dietro la nuca. (*Le novelle*, 158–59)

> [But the sisters considered the woman's imbecility and infirmity one of those supreme proofs of martyrdom to which the Lord calls the elect in order to sanctify and glorify them afterwards in Paradise, and they surrounded the idiot with veneration and care. In the summer of 1881 the signs of approaching death appeared. Consumed and scarred, that miserable body no longer retained anything human. Slow deformations had vitiated the posture of her limbs; tumors fat as apples sprouted on her side, on her shoulder, at the back of her head.]

Do we read *idiota* as Dostoevskian or assume that it carries the negative connotations of common parlance? The "signs of death" which appear on the virgin's body, in lieu of the possible "signs of martyrdom," seem to point in a Lombrosian direction. Yet even the demystifying Lombrosian stance is not as firm as it might be, for D'Annunzio could well have adopted the Flaubertian strategy of "Un coeur simple" and, rather than dispensing with Anna's beloved tortoise, made it an object of idolatry like Félicité's parrot.

What, then, do we make of these two tales? "La vergine Orsola," insofar as it is in complementary contrast with Andrea Sperelli's convalescence, is less problematic than "La vergine Anna." As a portrayal of convalescence as the bed of an "anticonversion," "La vergine Orsola," in a rhetorical sense, had to exist. The scene of convalescence is given a Lombrosian (and early Freudian) inflection that overturns the terms of the Baudelairean rhetoric. The topos of conversion evokes its dialectical counterpart, perversion, and convalescence becomes the ground for both conversion and perversion in D'Annunzio's works. "La vergine Anna" cannot be inserted into this framework; not only is convalescence not thematized, but neither a dramatic conversion nor an introduction to perversion occurs in the story. Anna's life is a series of illnesses and traumas, none of which is specifically sexual. As in Frau Emmy von N.'s account of her life, this version of Anna's biography appears to have been edited *in usum delphini*.[12] But from the tension between the narrator's adherence to the nun's interpretation of Anna's attacks and the narrator's demystifying "Lombrosian" moments, there arises a hint of a third interpretation: this, too, is the tale of a conversion, but the conversion here enacted is *hysterical* conversion. Anna exhibits symptoms that also characterize Freud and Breuer's *Fräulein und Frauen:* like Miss Lucy R., Anna has olfactory hallucinations; like Fräulein Anna O. and Frau Emmy von N., the virgin Anna's speech is disturbed and distorted; like Fräulein Elizabeth von R., Anna assumes positions that are iconic of her psychic condition:

> Come l'inferma entrava nell'estasi catalettica, i preludii vaghi dell'organo rapivano gli animi delle religiose in una sfera superiore. Il lume delle lampade si diffondeva fievole dall'alto, dando un'incertitudine aerea e quasi una morente dolcezza all'apparenza delle cose. A un punto l'organo taceva. La respirazione dell'inferma diveniva più profonda; le braccia le si

12. "It has also struck me that amongst all the intimate information given me by the patient there was a complete absence of the sexual element, which is, after all, more liable than any other to provide occasion for traumas. It is impossible that her excitations in this field can have left no traces whatsoever; what I was allowed to hear was no doubt an *editio in usum delphini* (a bowdlerized edition) of her life story" (Freud-Breuer, 103).

distendevano così che nei polsi scarnificati i tendini vibravano simili alle corde di uno strumento. Poi, d'un tratto, l'inferma balzava in piedi, incrociava le braccia sul petto, restando nell'atteggiamento mistico delle cariatidi d'un battistero. (*Le novelle,* 158)

[As the sick woman entered into cataleptic ecstasy, vague preludes on the organ lifted the souls of the nuns to a higher sphere. The light of the lamps spread dimly from above and gave an airy uncertainty and almost a dying sweetness to the appearance of things. At a certain point the organ fell silent. The sick woman breathed more deeply; her arms were stretched out so that the tendons in her emaciated wrists vibrated like the strings of an instrument. Then suddenly the sick woman would jump to her feet, cross her arms on her breast and stand in the mystical position of the caryatids of a baptistry.]

Anna's religious devotion is manifested through her body and made visible by a sort of hysterical conversion. The position described, in fact, recalls one of the common postures assumed by hysterics as recorded by Charcot.[13] As Jacques Goudet puts it, "La vergine Anna" is "a beautiful study of mystical hysteria."[14] This series of "coincidences"—fräuleins and virgins as objects of study, similar symptomatologies, a handbook hysterical posture—adds up to more than superficial similarity. The rhetoric of sickness D'Annunzio employs is not, I propose, reducible to "illness as metaphor" but instead implies a theory of the relationship between body and psyche. Physiological disease is adopted as a form of presentation of psychic contents, a rhetorical strategy chosen from among other possible modes of presentation of mental events. This literary choice has, however, epistemological implications: the body so described has no other outlet for the expression of psychic events. This mode

13. See, in particular, the "attitude passionelle" labeled "crucifiement" in Georges Didi-Huberman's study of *L'iconographie de la Salpêtrière,* titled *Invention de l'hysterie: Charcot et l'iconographie de la Salpêtrière* (Paris: Macula, 1982), fig. 7, p. 262.
14. Jacques Goudet, *D'Annunzio romanziere* (Florence: Olschki, 1976), 23.

of expression differs radically from the mode attributed to the male convalescents of Chapter 2, for this "speaker" is neither aware that a message is being transmitted nor fluent in the language employed. The choice of this mode of "speech" is, according to Freud and Breuer, precisely the hysteric's unconscious choice. The woman's body is spoken through once again, but it is not she who speaks; she is not a ventriloquist but a hysteric.

This is a "strong" reading of "La vergine Anna" and might provoke equally strong objections. Let me add, then, to the accumulation of "coincidences" around Signorina Anna's case. D'Annunzio places his female subject in an archaic context; despite the story's fictional collocation in the nineteenth century, it seems to take place, as Mario Ricciardi has noted, in a peasant community outside of history.[15] There are no workers here, no invasion of industrialization as in the works of the naturalist and verist schools, but instead the story of a "visionary" virgin rewarded with veneration. D'Annunzio's archaizing choice brings to mind not only Lombroso but also a more recent discussion of female sexuality which sees in cases of "mystical hysteria" a paradigm of female sexuality: Jacques Lacan's discussion of female sexuality, which radiates from an image of Saint Theresa, whom Breuer had called the "patron saint of hysteria" (Freud-Breuer, 232).[16] And though Freud makes it quite clear that he is dealing with solid, bourgeois gentlewomen (except in the case of the peasant Katharina), his techniques and language betray an archaizing tendency. The hysteric's body speaks in an ancient tongue, pictographic script, and the techniques used to test her are those established by the witch-hunters of the *Malleus malefi-*

15. Ricciardi, in *Coscienza e struttura nella prosa di D'Annunzio* (Turin: Giappichelli, 1970), discusses the "mythic dimension" in which *Terra vergine* and *Le novelle della Pescara* are situated: "It is here in the emergence of local history, in the 'barbaric' exaltation of primitive and immutable types of the Abruzzi region, that the last step of a gnoseological commitment is taken; in this direction, a polemical intent is confirmed, an intent to rediscover the actual social reality, ignored but now declined to the limits of the most brazen exoticism, by defining its traits according to a realism so extreme as to bring these types to a mythical zone, without time or history" (25).

16. I refer to Jacques Lacan, *Séminaire, livre 20—encore,* ed. Jacques-Alain Miller (Paris: Seuil, 1975).

carum. When Freud pinches the numb limbs of Elizabeth von R., he imitates those witch-hunters who likewise pricked and probed the unfeeling bodies of accused witches to discover not hysterogenic zones, but the paw print of the devil.[17]

As in Lombroso's studies, in which woman is placed several rungs lower than man on the evolutionary scale, Freud and Breuer and D'Annunzio place her "outside of history" or in archaic contexts in order to analyze her. Such an archaizing contextualization might, of course, be interpreted as an attempt to reread history. Indeed, the historically "progressive" move of positivism was to reinterpret mysticism and witchcraft as categories of experience deriving from the body rather than from the spirit. Witches and mystics became mere victims of normal neuroses. Yet in Freud and Breuer's and D'Annunzio's texts, naturalistic representation coexists uneasily with reverberations from contemporary psychohistorical investigations. Archaizing contextualizations appear to limit and mystify the relationship of the female body to thought, for they raise the positivistic reinterpretation to a general statement on the female condition and limit woman's "thought" (for mystical experience can be considered a form of thought) to the production of corporeal symptoms.

---

17. The alienists themselves were well aware of the source of this technique. B. A. Morel, in *Traité des maladies mentales* (Paris: Librairies Victor Masson, 1860), describes the witch-hunter's technique: "The slightest spot on the skin was probed with a needle. If the pricking caused no painful feeling, if it provoked neither cries nor movement, then the poor sick person was a sorcerer and condemned to be burned alive. If, on the contrary, he felt the prick, he was acquitted: Satan had not left his paw print" (320). Lombroso, with his usual nonchalance, spells out the rest: "La grande prova, infatti, di colpa in stregoneria erano i cosidetti segni della zampa del diavolo, i punti della pelle che si potevano pungere senza dolore ed emorragia; si trattava evidentemente di quelle zone anestetiche così caratteristiche dell'isterismo" ["In fact, the great proof of guilt in witchcraft were the so-called marks of the devil's paw, the points on the skin that could be pricked without pain or bleeding; clearly they were those anesthetic zones so characteristic of hysteria"] (*La donna delinquente,* 203). The techniques of trial and torture are set out in Heinrich Kramer and James Sprenger, *Malleus maleficarum,* trans. Montague Summers (1508; London: Arrow Books, 1971). See also, for a discussion of the relationship between demonology and hysteria, Ilza Veith, *Hysteria: The History of a Disease* (Chicago: University of Chicago Press, 1965).

The Influenza of Baudelaire

Far from refuting the medicolegal diagnosis that hoped for their early demise, the decadents incorporated it into their writings, once again transforming insult into a mark of distinction. It is here that the other face of Baudelaire—Baudelaire's illness as text— emerges, for this aspect of Baudelairean "influenza" is filtered through the Lombrosian rhetoric. This appearance of a Lombrosian rhetoric in the description of upper-class protagonists has often been read as merely a response to naturalism. Marc Fumaroli, in his preface to *A rebours,* suggests parodic intentions:

> There is something willingly false and pastiched about the naturalist elements imbricated in this strange monster. Such is the case of the "medical report" which Huysmans provides for Des Esseintes: his "heredity," emphatically invoked in order to "explain" his "degeneration," his "neurosis," described by dint of technical terms and based on authoritative scientific works. That, at least, is what Huysmans asserted to Zola in order to reassure him. In the episode, recounted with great seriousness, of the liquid meals administered by clysters, the "clinical case" aspect of Des Esseintes openly becomes a big joke, worthy of the *Malade imaginaire.*[18]

If indeed the clinical aspect of Huysmans's novel is a parody of naturalism, a barb aimed at Zola, it is also an integral part of decadent narrative. It might, in fact, be more appropriate to speak of a polemical response rather than parody, for while naturalism speaks from the island of normalcy, decadentism speaks through that pathological other which naturalism paternalistically describes. The distance that separates the naturalistic narrator from his pathological subjects is replaced by an identification with pathology and degeneracy.

Yet the "naturalism" of the decadent text is applied in a nonnaturalistic, delirious fashion, for the pathology with which the decadents identify is of a quite specific sort. Des Esseintes, for example,

18. Marc Fumaroli, Préface to J. K. Huysmans, *A rebours,* ed. Fumaroli (Paris: Gallimard, 1977), 22.

is an ardent admirer not only of Baudelaire's writings but also of his symptoms. His enfeebled digestive system, his aural and olfactory hallucinations, his nightmarish visions of syphilis all recall Baudelaire's disease as annotated both by the poet himself and in contemporary medical accounts. It is as though literary inheritance were figured as biological inheritance of the disease of the literary father. Influence truly becomes influenza.

Huysmans's fellow decadents were quick to point out the spiritual similarities between Huysmans and his idol Baudelaire. Barbey d'Aurevilly wrote apropos of *A rebours:*

> Eh bien, un jour, je défiai l'originalité de Baudelaire de recommencer les *Fleurs du mal* et de faire un pas de plus dans le sens épuisé du blasphème. Je serais bien capable de porter à l'auteur d'*A rebours* le même défi: "Après les *Fleurs du mal*— dis-je à Baudelaire,—il ne vous reste plus, logiquement, que la bouche d'un pistolet ou les pieds de la croix." Baudelaire choisit les pieds de la croix.
> Mais l'auteur d'*A Rebours* les choisira-t-il?[19]

> [Well, one day I challenged Baudeliare's originality to begin the *Fleurs du mal* over again and to take another step along the worn-out path of blasphemy. I would be quite capable of similarly challenging the author of *A Rebours:* "After the *Fleurs du mal*," I said to Baudelaire, "you logically have only one choice left: either the mouth of a pistol or the feet of the cross." Baudelaire chose the feet of the cross. But will the author of *A rebours* choose them?]

Barbey d'Aurevilly succeeded in predicting the future, for Huysmans did indeed choose the foot of the cross later in his career. But in 1884, the year *A rebours* was published, the association of the two is prompted by both mystical and medical similarities: the blasphemous Huysmans recalls the satanic Baudelaire; Des Esseintes the convalescent recalls the dying Baudelaire. That Baude-

---

19. Jules Barbey d'Aurevilly, *Le roman contemporain* (Geneva: Slatkine Reprints, 1968), 273; originally published as *"A rebours"* in *Le Constitutionnel,* 28 July 1884.

laire's unfortunate end was a continual source of fascination to the decadents is attested by Maurice Barrès's essay of the same year. In "La folie de Baudelaire," Barrès commemorates the afflicted poet with a rundown of his symptoms. Barbey d'Aurevilly's bons mots are fresh in Barres's memory, and the portrait he presents seems to become a double exposure in which both Baudelaire's and Des Esseintes's features can be glimpsed. If Barbey d'Aurevilly predicted Huysmans's spiritual future, then Barrès predicts Des Esseintes's medical future:

"Se suicider ou se faire chrétien!" Le poète n'eut pas à choisir. Depuis des années dejà son organisme affolé se refusait au service quotidien. La paralysie l'envahissait. A l'âge de quarante-six ans le 31 août 1867, Charles Baudelaire expira à Bruxelles, où son inquiétude cherchait quelque repos. Il était de sa destinée de ne le trouver qu'en la tombe. Depuis un an déjà l'aphasie liait sa langue. Qui sait si l'intelligence elle-même ne sombre point dans cette aventure. Des amis vinrent sur son cadavre encore tiède affirmer son esprit lucide dans l'agonie dernière. Jusqu'au cercueil ils soutinrent pieusement cette tête vide qui ballottait de-ci de-là.[20]

["Commit suicide or become Christian!" The poet had no choice. For years his maddened organism had resisted daily service. Paralysis had invaded it. At the age of forty-six, 31 August 1867, Charles Baudelaire expired in Brussels, where his restlessness had sought some repose. It was his fate to find it only in the grave. Aphasia had tied his tongue for a year. Who knows if the mind itself does not founder when it comes to such a pass. Friends gathered around his still-warm corpse to affirm that his spirit was still lucid in the final agony. To the very coffin, they piously held up the empty head that bobbed from side to side.]

This mythification of Baudelaire's final years emphasizes three symptoms which will recur in medical reports as well: paralysis,

20. Maurice Barrès, "La folie de Charles Baudelaire," in *L'oeuvre de Maurice Barrès*, ed. Philippe Barrès (Paris: Au Club de l'Honnête Homme, 1965), 1:401, originally published in *Les Taches d'Encre*, 5 November 1884.

aphasia, and imbecility. The horrifying appeal of these symptoms to a writer's imagination is clear; they are, all three, physical impediments to the writer's craft. For the decadents, for whom Baudelaire stands as legitimating father, the threat is even greater, if less rational, than for the writer in general. Ideological sympathy threatens to become physiological similarity. It is precisely this threat that D'Annunzio's Baudelairean convalescent experiences in the moment in which he is most Baudelairean, in which he is closest to Constantin Guys.

Having just rediscovered "l'Arte . . . l'Amante fedele," Andrea Sperelli also discovers the shadow of Baudelaire's final years:

> La lenta decadenza dell'ingegno può anche essere inconsciente: qui sta il terribile. L'Artista che a poco a poco perde le sue facoltà non si accorge della sua debolezza progressiva, poiché insieme con la potenza di produrre e di riprodurre lo abbandona anche il giudizio critico, il criterio. Egli non distingue più i difetti dell'opera sua; non sa che la sua opera è cattiva o mediocre; s'illude; crede che il suo quadro, che la sua statua, che il suo poema sieno nelle leggi dell'arte mentre son fuori. Qui sta il terribile. L'artista colpito nell'intelletto può non aver conscienza della propria imbecillità, come il pazzo non ha conscienza della propria aberrazione. E allora? Fu pel convalescente una specie di panico. (*Il piacere*, 147)

> [The slow decay of the mind can also be unconscious: that is the terrible thing about it. The Artist who loses his faculties little by little is unaware of his progressive weakness, for he loses not only the power to produce and reproduce but also his critical judgment, his criterion. He no longer discerns the defects of his work; he does not know that his work is bad or mediocre; he deludes himself; he believes that his painting or his statue or his poem is within laws of art when it is instead outside them. That is the frightful thing. The artist stricken in his intellect may not be aware of his own imbecility, just as the madman is unaware of his own aberration. And then what? This was a sort of panic for the convalescent.]

It is not the language of this passage which is Lombrosian but the fact that a fear of imbecility accompanies Sperelli's discovery of his identity as an artist. It is as though Sperelli in miming the Baudelairean convalescent risks miming the biographical Baudelaire. The Lombrosian rhetoric of sickness aims precisely to reduce all signs to symptoms of somatic illness, to read literary works as physiological tics. Constantin Guys and Charles Baudelaire represent divergent and contrasting models of the relationship between the (upper-class male) body and thought. Guys's eternal convalescence makes it possible for him to become an artist, a manipulator and producer of signs. Baudelaire's sickness instead represents an unconscious production of symptoms, an inability to distinguish between symptoms produced by the body and signs produced by the intellect. These two rhetorics—that of convalescence as the scene of artistic creation, of conversion to art, and that of sickness as the production of mere symptoms, of hysterical conversion—come perilously close to collision. The separate tracks of these rhetorics meet and conflict in Andrea Sperelli; as he rediscovers his capacity to produce signs, he fears that those signs might instead be nothing more than corporeal symptoms.

The narrator of *L'Innocente,* Tullio Hermil, is similarly haunted by this specter of a Baudelaire (or, indeed, a Maupassant or a Nietzsche) overcome by paralysis and aphasia.[21] Hermil, too, is convalescent, though no physiological disease or wound provides an alibi for his rebirth. In the opening section of the novel, a sort of *incipit* that precedes the first enumerated chapter, illness appears as a metaphor for a life of perversion:

La mia triste passione per Teresa Raffo divenne sempre più esclusiva, occupò tutte le mie facoltà, non mi diede un'ora di tregua. Io era veramente un ossesso, un uomo invaso da una diabolica follia, corroso da un morbo ignoto e spaventevole.[22]

21. Nietzsche and Maupassant both suffered from this aspect of Baudelairean *influenza*. It was in 1889 in Lombroso's Turin that Nietzsche crossed the threshold into madness and in 1889 that Maupassant began his descent toward madness and his eventual death in 1893. For biographical details, see Walter Kaufmann, *Nietzsche: Philosopher, Psychologist, Antichrist* (Princeton: Princeton University Press, 1968); and Michael G. Lerner, *Maupassant* (London: George Allen and Unwin, 1975).
22. Gabriele D'Annunzio, *L'Innocente,* in *Prose di romanzi,* 1:415.

[My sad passion for Teresa Raffo became ever more exclusive; it occupied all my faculties and gave me not a single hour of peace. I was truly an obsessed man, a man possessed by a diabolical madness, corroded by an unknown and frightful malady.]

His, he tells us, is an entirely spiritual convalescence, a conversion from the "sozzura fallica" ["phallic filth"], represented by Teresa Raffo, to a purer mode of being:

Le grandi malattie dell'anima come quelle del corpo rinovellano l'uomo; e le convalescenze spirituali non sono meno soavi e meno miracolose di quelle fisiche. Davanti a un arbusto fiorito, davanti a un ramo coperto di minute gemme, davanti a un rampollo nato su un vecchio tronco quasi estinto, davanti alla più umile fra le grazie della terra, davanti alla più modesta fra le trasfigurazioni della primavera, io mi soffermavo semplice, candido, attonito! (*L'Innocente*, 423)

[Great illnesses of the soul, like those of the body, renew man, and spiritual convalescences are not less sweet or less miraculous than physical ones. Before a flowering shrub, before a branch covered with tiny buds, before a shoot born from an old and almost extinct trunk, before the most humble of the earth's beauties, before the most modest of spring's transfigurations, I stopped, simple, pure, astonished!]

Like Sperelli, Hermil discovers the liberating tabula rasa of the convalescent, and once again a Lombrosian shadow appears in the context of a Baudelairean convalescence, though here it appears projected upon Hermil's rival and double, Filippo Arborio. Hermil, himself expert in the art of seduction, describes his wife's seducer in terms that suggest a self-portrait (and in fact anticipate the terms with which D'Annunzio's biographers and critics will describe D'Annunzio himself):

Filippo Arborio, esperto, avendo indovinato la special condizione fisica della donna ch'egli voleva possedere, s'era servito del metodo più conveniente e più sicuro, che è questo: —

parlare di idealità, di zone superiori, di alleanze mistiche, ed occupare nel tempo medesimo le mani alla scoperta d'altri misteri; unire insomma un brano di pura eloquenza a una delicata manomessione. (*L'Innocente*, 510–11)

[Experienced in such matters, Filippo Arborio had divined the special physical condition of the women he wanted to possess, and he had adopted the most appropriate and surest method, which is this: —speak of the ideal, of higher realms, of mystical alliances, and at the same time occupy one's hands in the discovery of other mysteries. In short, unite a passage of pure eloquence with a delicate laying on of hands.]

Projected upon Arborio, sickness becomes murder by wish fulfillment; Hermil wishes a tragic end upon his wife's lover moments before he receives confirmation of its fulfillment from an albino bookseller:

E m'augurai che si trattasse d'una di quelle terribili malattie del midollo spinale o della sostanza cerebrale, che conducono un uomo alle infime degradazioni, all'idiotismo, alle più tristi forme della follia e quindi alla morte. Le nozioni apprese dai libri di scienza, i ricordi di una visita a un manicomio, le imagini anche più precise lasciatemi impresse dal caso speciale di un mio amico, del povero Spinelli, ora mi tornavano alla memoria rapidamente. E rivedevo il povero Spinelli seduto su la gran poltrona di cuoio rosso, pallido d'un pallor terreo, con tutti i lineamenti della faccia irrigiditi, con la bocca dilatata e aperta, piena di saliva e d'un balbettio incomprensibile. (*L'Innocente*, 557)

[And I hoped that it was one of those terrible diseases of the spinal cord or of the cerebral substance that reduce a man to the lowest degradations, to idiocy, to the most pitiful forms of madness and finally to death. Notions learned from scientific books, memories of a visit to an insane asylum, the even more precise images that had impressed themselves upon me in the special case of a friend of mine, poor Spinelli, now all rushed back into my memory. And I saw again poor Spinelli, seated in a large red leather armchair, pale with an ashen pallor, with all the lines of his face rigidifed, his mouth open and gaping, full of saliva and an incomprehensible babble.]

The paronomasia of "Spinelli," who appears only in these few pages, with "Sperelli" is irresistible, not only because Sperelli's fear becomes Spinelli's reality but because Spinelli is associated by medical analogy with Filippo Arborio, whose forthcoming novel was to have been titled *Turris eburnea*. It is as though the hero of the first book of the *Romanzi della Rosa* returned in the second, having in the meantime dedicated a novel to Maria Ferres, *turris eburnea*, and contracted the feared disease. This connection is, of course, not systematic but part of the rhetoric that also links Hermil to Arborio; Hermil's confession is presumably a revelation of his crime, "il mio segreto," which echoes the title of Arborio's latest novel, *Il segreto*—precisely the book that the pale clerk offers him in this scene. Arborio is both a literary and a sexual rival, and his sickness precludes the necessity of homicide; it is in itself a homicide by what Freud will call animistic thinking:

Pensavo: "Ho tutto da guadagnare. Se avessi un duello con un avversario così celebre, se lo ferissi gravemente, se l'uccidessi, il fatto, certo, non rimarrebbe segreto; correrebbe su tutte le bocche, sarebbe divulgato, commentato da tutte le gazzette. E potrebbe anche venire in chiaro la causa vera del duello! Invece questa malattia provvidenziale mi salva da ogni pericolo, da ogni fastidio, da ogni pettegolezzo. Io posso ben rinunziare a una voluttà sanguinaria, a un castigo inflitto con la mia mano (e sono poi certo dell'esito?), quando so paralizzato dalla malattia, ridotto all'impotenza l'uomo che detesto. Ma la notizia sarà vero? E se si trattasse di un disturbo transitorio?" Mi venne una buona idea. Saltai in una vettura e mi fece condurre alla libreria dell'editore. Nella strada consideravo mentalmente (con un voto sincero) i due disturbi cerebrali più terribili per un uomo di lettere, per un artefice della parola, per uno stilista: —l'afasia e l'agrafia. E avevo la visione fantastica dei sintomi. (*L'Innocente*, 557–58)

[I thought: "I have everything to gain. If I were to duel such a famous adversary, if I were to wound him seriously or kill him, the fact would certainly not remain secret. It would spread quickly by word-of-mouth and would be in all the papers. The true cause of the duel might even come out! And instead this providential sickness saves me from all perils, from all annoyances, and from all the gossip. I can surely renounce a bloody pleasure, a punishment inflicted by my own hand (and am I so sure of the outcome?), when I know that the man I detest is paralyzed by his disease and reduced to impotence. But can this news be true? And what if it were a transitory disturbance?" A good idea occurred to me. I jumped into a carriage and had it take me to his editor's bookstore. On the way I mentally pictured (with a sincere vow) the two cerebral disturbances most terrible for a man of letters, for the craftsman of the word, for a stylist: aphasia and agraphia. And I had an imaginary vision of the symptoms.]

Later in the novel, Hermil will exploit this intuition of the exculpatory possibilities of disease in matters of murder; infanticide by induced pneumonia is, of course, the crime to which Hermil ostensibly confesses. Here he limits himself to wishing upon his double Baudelaire's symptoms—paralysis, aphasia, and one of Lombroso's favorite categories in *La donna delinquente, agrafia*. The bookseller supplies both confirmation and nomenclature of the hoped-for disease:

> —Il romanziere è molto malato!
> —Malato! Di che male?
> —D'una paralisi bulbare progressiva—rispose l'albino distaccando le parole terribili l'una dall'altra, con una certa affettazione di saccente. "Ah, il male di Giulio Spinelli!"
> (*L'Innocente*, 558–59)

> ["The novelist is very sick!"
> "Sick! What does he have?"
> "A progressive paralysis of the medulla oblongata," replied the albino, separating the terrible words with a certain scientific affectation. "Oh, The same illness that Giulio Spinelli had!"]

Tullio and the bookseller then consult medical texts to ascertain the incurability of Arborio's condition, just as D'Annunzio claimed to have consulted medical texts in the researching and writing of *L'Innocente*.[23] Whether or not D'Annunzio consulted *Genio e follia* (1882) or the then recent rewrite of that volume, *L'uomo di genio* (1892), the diagnosis echoes Lombroso's diagnosis of Baudelaire: "finì colla paralisi progressiva degli alienati" ["ended with the progressive paralysis of *alienati*"].[24]

At this point, both Lombroso and Baudelaire are clearly metonymies; Baudelaire could well be a number of Lombroso's *alienati*, Lombroso, a number of fellow alienists. What is important here is the appearance of Lombrosian alienist language and symptomatologies. Tullio Hermil, in fact, describes himself as an alienist would describe an *alienato:*

> Quante volte io, ideologo e analista e sofista in epoca di decadenza, m'ero compiaciuto d'essere il discendente di quel Raimondo Hermil de Penedo che alla Goletta operò prodigi di valore e di ferocia sotto gli occhi di Carlo Quinto! Lo sviluppo eccessivo della mia intelligenza e la mia *multanimità* non avevano potuto modificare il fondo della mia sostanza, il substrato nascosto in cui erano inscritti tutti i caratteri ereditarii della mia razza. In mio fratello, organismo equilibrato, il

23. In her preface to the 1976 Oscar Mondadori edition of *L'Innocente,* Maria Teresa Giannelli states that, in his correspondence with his French translator, Georges Hérelle, D'Annunzio claims to have researched the symptoms of the adulterine child's illness and death (23). She does not, however, cite the letter involved, and it does not appear in the collection of letters published as *Gabriele D'Annunzio à Georges Hérelle: Correspondance,* ed. Guy Tosi (Paris: Denoël, 1946). But in his introductory note to that collection, Tosi recounts an episode from Hérelle's manuscript "Notolette dannunziane" which seems to corroborate Giannelli's reference. D'Annunzio happens upon a child suffering from croup, and tries to put his medical studies to use: "J'avais essayé, sans succès, de le soulager à l'aide du peu de connaissances médicales que j'avais acquises lorsque je faisais des études pour la description de la mort du petit Raymond dans *L'Innocente*" ["I tried, unsuccessfully, to relieve it with the help of the little medical knowledge I had acquired when I did research for the description of the death of Raimondo in *L'Innocente*"] (33).

24. Cesare Lombroso, *L'uomo di genio in rapporto alla psichiatria, alla storia ed all'estetica,* 6th ed. (Turin: Fratelli Bocca, 1894), 101.

pensiero s'accompagnava sempre all'opera; in me il pensiero predominava ma senza distruggere le mie facoltà di azione che anzi non di rado si esplicavano con una straordinaria potenza. Io ero insomma un violento e un appassionato consciente, nel quale l'ipertrofia di alcuni centri cerebrali rendeva impossibile la coordinazione necessaria alla vita normale dello spirito. Lucidissimo sorvegliatore di me stesso, avevo tutti gli impeti delle nature primitive indisciplinabili. Più di una volta io ero stato tentato da improvvise suggestioni delittuose. Più d'una volta ero rimasto sorpreso dall'insurrezione spontanea d'un istinto crudele. (*L'Innocente,* 514–15)

[How often I, ideologue and analyst and sophist in an epoch of decadence, had prided myself on being the descendant of that Raimondo Hermil de Penedo who had worked miracles of valor and ferocity before the eyes of Charles V! The excessive development of my intelligence and my *many-souledness* had not been able to modify the foundation of my substance, the hidden substratum in which all the hereditary characteristics of my race were inscribed. In my brother, a balanced organism, thought and action were always linked; in me, thought predominated, yet without destroying my faculties of action, which in fact often unfolded with extraordinary power. In short, I was a violent and passionate, conscious man, in whom the hypertrophy of certain cerebral centers rendered impossible the coordination necessary to the normal life of the spirit. An extremely lucid observer of myself, I had all the impulses of undisciplinable, primitive natures. More than once I had been tempted by sudden criminal ideas. More than once I had been surprised by the spontaneous insurrection of a cruel instinct.]

Lombroso appears once again *in filigrana,* for Hermil attributes to himself the pathological symptoms of genius and a concomitant tendency toward "follia morale." Both the technical terms and the general outline of Hermil's character are Lombrosian:

Mancare di talento, o meglio di buon senso, di senso comune, è questo uno dei caratteri speciali del genio, e che ne sigillano la nevrosi, la psicosi, indicando che l'ipertrofia di alcuni centri psichici è, come diciamo tecnicamente, compensata da parziali atrofie di altri. (*L'uomo di genio,* xxi)

[To lack talent, or better, to lack good sense or common sense, is one of the special characteristics of genius; it is the stamp of neurosis and psychosis and indicates that the hypertrophy of certain psychic centers is, technically speaking, compensated by partial atrophies of others.]

Hermil's supposed analytic abilities and extraordinary lucidity are, for a Lombrosian, further proof that Hermil is a pathological case. Lombroso comments, apropos of the writings of "average" degenerates:

Ogni numero, quasi, di questi curiosi diari, portava in se, e risuggellava la dimostrazione di quella tesi, creduta per tanto tempo un bislacco paradosso, e riesciva a convincere i più: quanto poco nell'alienato s'avveri di quel caotico e assurdo che le menti volgari vi appiccicano, e come anzi spesso, l'alienazione dia luogo ad una, non ordinaria, lucidezza di mente. (*Genio e follia,* Premessa)

[Almost every one of these strange diaries carried within it and reconfirmed the demonstration of our thesis, and managed to convince most people of what had long been considered a quaint paradox: very rarely does one find the chaotic and absurd elements that the man on the street attaches to the *alienato,* but on the contrary, alienation often gives rise to an extraordinary lucidity of mind.]

D'Annunzio did his homework so well that the alienists themselves recognized their theories in Tullio Hermil. Enrico Ferri concluded, not surprisingly, that Hermil was a born criminal.[25]

25. Enrico Ferri describes Tullio Hermil thus: "Tullio Hermil, in Gabriele D'Annunzio's *Innocente,* is one of those elegantly dressed scoundrels whom one meets on the sidewalks of big cities, a born criminal on account of the congenital atrophy of the moral sense and corresponding hypertrophy of the ego, especially of the sexual ego—who does not of course resort to the ingenuous and primitive method of poison or knife in order to kill a human creature but who is not for this any less degenerate and perverse." Enrico Ferri, *I delinquenti nell'arte,* 2d ed. (Turin: UTET, 1926), 127.

But if Tullio Hermil describes himself as a Lombrosian might have, D'Annunzio reads Hermil's symptoms as Freud might have, reads them by presenting a first-person narrative whose narrator protests too much that he is an acute and accurate analyst of himself. Here symptoms do not appear on the body, as was the case with the virgin Anna; they manifest themselves in discourse. The unreliable narrator's moments of self-analysis assert themselves as the metalanguage that "explains" the flow of his confession. But if instead we reverse the terms and read the confession as the metalanguage that interprets those moments of self-definition, we discover that Hermil's Lombrosian professions are undermined by the rhetorical strategies employed in the text.

The opening lines of the novel put into question the status of this "confession":

> Andare davanti al giudice, dirgli: "Ho commesso un delitto. Quella povera creatura non sarebbe morta se io non l'avessi uccisa. Io Tullio Hermil, io stesso l'ho uccisa. Ho premeditato l'assassinio, nella mia casa. L'ho compiuto con una perfetta lucidità di conscienza, esattamente, nella massima sicurezza. Poi ho seguitato a vivere col mio segreto nella mia casa, un anno intero, fino ad oggi. Oggi è l'anniversario. Eccomi nelle vostre mani. Ascoltatemi. Giudicatemi." Posso andare davanti al giudice, posso parlargli così?
>
> Non posso né voglio. La giustizia degli uomini non mi tocca. Nessun tribunale della terra saprebbe giudicarmi.
>
> Eppure bisogna che io mi accusi, che io mi confessi. Bisogna che io riveli il mio segreto a qualcuno.
>
> A CHI? (*L'Innocente,* 370)

[To go before the judge and say to him: "I committed a crime. That poor creature would not be dead if I had not killed it. I myself, Tullio Hermil, killed it. I premeditated the assassination in my own house. I carried it out with perfect lucidity of consciousness, precisely, in the greatest security. Then I continued to live with my secret in my house, an entire year up to today. Today is the anniversary. Here I am in your hands. Listen to me. Judge me." Can I go before the judge, can I speak to him thus?

I cannot, nor do I wish to. The justice of men does not touch me. No court on earth would know how to judge me.
And yet I must accuse myself, I must confess. I must reveal my secret to someone.
TO WHOM?]

A *confessione* may be an admission of guilt, a declaration of illegal or immoral acts committed; it may (in the reflexive form *confessarsi*) be the manifestation of one's sins in the Christian sacrament of Confession; it may also be a profession of a faith, a doctrine, a religion. In the case of a confessional (Christian) text like Saint Augustine's, these differing meanings presumably form a seamless whole: a "profession" of Christian faith requires a "confession" of one's sins, a confession of guilt and immoral acts. But the possibility of a secular rift between "confession" and "profession" presents itself: one might "confess" to a crime but at the same time deny that any "crime" has been committed according to one's own doctrines. This, in fact, seems to be Hermil's strategy: his admission of guilt is merely a sample of a possible confession, closed off by quotation marks, and the profession that follows negates that sample. Not only can he not say "I, Tullio Hermil, committed a crime," but he denies the very possibility of a confession by denying the existence of a qualified judge. Or at least, one might argue, of a secular judge, for the only form of *confessare* the narrator uses is the reflexive, sacramental form: "bisogna...che io mi confessi." "A CHI?" comes the response. The question puts into question even the possibility of a sovereign judge and hence the validity of confession itself. What is left is only desacralizing profession,[26] an anticonfession, or a confession through negation. It would appear to be all three. The very title of the novel contains a hint of this desacralization, for while *L'Innocente* refers, we learn toward the end

26. Luchino Visconti's film *L'Innocente* in fact presents Hermil as more of a "profess-or" than confessor. Though it is true that Visconti's representation of Hermil as a mixture of the biographical D'Annunzio, a two-bit stereotypical Nietzsche, and a nihilist is less than faithful to the novel, the opening frames of the film, with shots of the book itself as a hand leafs quickly through its pages (rather than, for example, a shot of the book as it is opened followed by a fade to the first scene of the film), suggest that Visconti's film does not attempt to "read" the novel and has dispensed with the very problem of fidelity.

of the novel, to the child after baptism, it also inevitably refers to the "profess-or" himself, "innocent" of crime. A liturgical scheme is invoked only to be desacralized: Easter become the occasion of the *resurrezione* of Tullio and Giuliana's "passion;" Christmas, the occasion of the child's death, rather than birth. Tullio and Giuliana read together poems from Verlaine's *Sagesse,* written as testimony to his conversion, precisely in the moment when Tullio is about (once again) to leave the *diritta via.* Still caught in the system it would degrade, a desacralizing profession is an anticonfession. And the form this anticonfession takes is a confession through negation: not "I did this and I did that," but "I did not do this, nor did I do that."

(De)negation is but one of the ways that unconscious material may make its way to consciousness, according to Freud.[27] The superlucid narrator is, in fact, at the mercy of mechanisms of the unconscious; displacement, condensation, and denegation are Hermil's true strategies. Condensation works primarily upon names: Giuliana, *la sorella,* comes to be identified with Costanza, the dead sister, through the transfer of the sister's name, "costanza," to Giuliana herself, "costantemente fedele," "la mia adorazione costante" (450) ["constantly faithful" "my constant adoration"]; "la sorella unica" ["the only sister"] becomes "la sorella, Unica" ["the sister, Unique"]. A particularly "dense" condensation occurs in the naming of the adulterine child, Raimondo, for Raimondo is, of course, the name of Hermil's father. By itself, such a naming could be simply a detail of sociological interest, but as we shall see, its insertion into the narrative justifies considering it an example of condensation.

The contrast between the *incipit* and the narration that "begins" with chapter 1 testifies to the presence of extensive displacement. Hermil begins his confession twice as he attempts to arrive at the "primo ricordo," which continues to elude him. A sort of chiastic tension is created between these two beginnings, for the traits that characterize Giuliana in the *incipit* characterize Hermil in the second "primo ricordo," and vice versa. It is Giuliana who is convalescent

27. See Sigmund Freud, "Negation," in *Standard Edition,* 19. The article is dated 1925. I use the term *denegation,* modeled on the French translation of *Verneinung* as *dénegation,* in order to mark this "negation" as Freudian.

in the *incipit* (she recovers from a gynecological operation), Giuliana who is faithful and pure, Guiliana who is sororal. In the second section, it is Tullio who is convalescent, Tullio who has become faithful and pure, Tullio whose fraternal role is emphasized in relation to his brother Federico. This exchange of qualities works both ways, for it is Tullio who is unfaithful in the *incipit,* unable to separate himself from the "imagine fallica, una sozzura" ["phallic image, a filthy thing"] (represented by Teresa Raffo), which had become his "morbo ignoto." In the second section, Giuliana's infidelity is revealed; the narrative focuses on Giuliana's "fallo," her sin, and the resultant pregnancy becomes Giuliana's "morbo."[28] This transfer of characteristics is a transference of guilt; attention is shifted from the narrator's infidelity to Giuliana's supposed affair. Such an exchange of qualities renders Hermil's "true confession" suspect and suggests that his narrative is a symptomatic one.

Suspicion mounts as our reading proceeds. The characters of *L'Innocente,* who are linked by sexual and familial relations, fall into three categories, each of which contains three characters: a triad of adult women comprising Giuliana, Hermil's mother, and Teresa Raffo; a group of adult men including Tullio, his brother Federico, and Arborio; and a trio of female children—Maria, Natalia, and Costanza, dead but ever-present to Hermil. In each group of three, the third member is present only as an absence: Teresa is referred to as "L'Assente" ["The Absent One"]; Costanza, Hermil's sister, is dead; Filippo Arborio, who is dying, is referred to as "L'Altro" ["The Other"]. In the group of women, Teresa and Hermil's mother are linked to Giuliana as representations of her maternal and erotic potentialities. In the triad of men, Federico seems to represent Tullio's "good" double, Arborio the seducer, his "bad" double. It is in the triad of children that a disturbance occurs, caused by the appearance of a fourth member: the adulterine child who bears the name of Hermil's father. This child must be eliminated because he belongs to too many categories, he is simply one too many: he is Giuliana's child, Arborio's progeny, Tullio's apparent heir, the bearer of Hermil's father's name. The play of similarities and doublings among these characters allows us to retell *L'Innocente* as a confession of a different series of crimes. We might, then, imagine

28. The consequences of the exchange of *falli* are discussed in Chapter 4.

a sort of ghost narrative in which Hermil would summarize his story in denegations and displacements. It might sound something like this: "It is not my mother but my wife who is with child in my mother's house. In any case, it was not I but Filippo Arborio who impregnated her. It was not I who killed that other but his disease. I merely desired his death, predicted his disease. It was not my son that I killed (and after all, it was pneumonia that killed him) but an intruder, an intruder with the name of my father but not my father." A series of displacements, of "rejection by projection," adds up to a confession through denegation: the narrator claims the child is not his own, just as Freud's dreamers will claim it is not their mother of whom they dream. But to what does Hermil confess? That Tullio is reenacting and reinterpreting a literary topos is made explicit by the text itself, as Tullio experiences a sense of déjà vu in deciding upon the murder method:

Certo, *mi ricordavo*. Era il ricordo d'una lettura lontana? Avevo trovato descritto in qualche libro un caso analogo? O qualcuno, un tempo, m'aveva narrato quel caso come occorso nella vita reale? Oppure quel sentimento del *ricordo* era illusorio, non era se non l'effetto d'una associazione d'idee misteriosa? Certo, mi pareva che il *mezzo* mi fosse stato suggerito da qualcuno estraneo. Mi pareva che qualcuno a un tratto fosse venuto a togliermi da ogni perplessità dicendomi: "*Bisogna che tu faccia così, come fece quell'altro nel tuo caso.*" Ma chi era quell'altro?...quell'uomo, il predecessore, m'era ignoto; e io non potevo associare a quella nozione le imagini relative senza mettere me stesso nel luogo di colui. Io dunque vedevo me stesso compiere quelle speciali azioni già compiute da un altro, imitare la condotta tenuta da un altro in un caso simile al mio. Il sentimento della spontaneità originale mi mancava. (*L'Innocente*, 617–18)

[Yes, *I remembered*. Was it the memory of something read long ago? Had I found an analogous case described in some book? Had someone, once, told me of that case as something that happened in real life? Or was this feeling of *remembrance* illusory, nothing but the effect of a mysterious association of ideas? It certainly seemed to me that the *means* had been suggested to me by someone else. It seemed that someone had suddenly come to me to relieve me of all doubts, by saying: *"You must do it in this way, as the other did in your case."* But who was *that other?* . . . that man, the predecessor, was unknown to me, and I could not associate that notion with the images relative to it without putting myself in his place. Thus I saw myself carrying out those special actions already carried out by another, I saw myself imitate the course of action taken by another in a case similar to my own. I had no feeling of original spontaneity.]

These "special actions" are, first and foremost, literary topoi: a narration, a book, a reading. At the same time as this passage describes Hermil trapped in a narration not his own, unable to read his symptoms as signs, it constitutes a set of instructions for reading the text: the narrative itself is a repetition. If Hermil cannot "remember" his predecessor, the reader can speculate, for it is as though three different but related mythological situations informed his confession: sibling rivalry with the son of the wife who so resembles Hermil's mother; an oedipal triangle in which the terms have undergone such distortion that Hermil becomes the apparent father of his father; another version of the Oedipus myth in which Hermil, however, plays the role not of Oedipus but of Laius as he exposes his feared and unwanted son to the elements.

Sibling rivalry is perhaps the least developed of these possibilities, thematized indirectly though nonetheless present. Arborio, Hermil's literary and sexual rival, is the author of a book that Hermil considers "fraternal," as well as the presumed father of the son who will threaten genealogical order. Hermil's unqualified praise for Federico, the Tolstoian brother, includes an evocation of primogeniture: "Avrei voluto essere da lui non soltanto amato ma dominato; avrei voluto cedere la primogenitura a lui più degno e star sommesso al suo consiglio, riguardarlo come la mia guida, obedirgli" (425) ["I would have liked to have been not only loved but also dominated by him. I would have liked to have given my primogeniture to him, more worthy than I, and to give myself over to his counsel, consider him my guide, obey him"]. Nothing of the kind happens, of course—not, that is, until Hermil contemplates the consequences of the birth of this child, "l'intruso che avrebbe portato il mio nome, che sarebbe stato il mio erede, che avrebbe usurpato le carezze di mia madre, delle mie figliuole, di mio fratello" (*L'Innocente*, 493) ["The intruder who would bear my name, who would be my heir, who would usurp the caresses of my mother, of my daughters, of my brother"].

> Giuliana dava alla luce un maschio, unico erede del nostro antico nome. Il figliuolo non mio cresceva, incolume, usurpava l'amore di mia madre, di mio fratello....diveniva capriccioso come un piccolo despota; s'impadroniva della mia casa. (*L'Innocente*, 539)

> Juliana gave birth to a boy, only heir to the family name. The son not mine grew, unharmed, and usurped the love of my mother, of my brother. . . . he became capricious, like a little despot; he became master of my house.

The child would "usurp" both the mother's love—that of *Hermil's* mother, not of Giuliana, Hermil's wife—and Hermil's property, *his* inheritance. As "unico erede" the child would indeed take away Hermil's primogeniture and thus might be said to figure as fraternal enemy.

The second possibility—that Hermil becomes the father of his father, the son of his son, and then acts out an oedipal narrative in disguised form—is perhaps the most obvious. Raimondo, the child who would usurp the mother's love, is none other than Raimondo, "l'uomo che mia madre amava" (569); in killing the son, Hermil kills the father.

The last possibility, however, suggests an interesting shift of focus in reading the Oedipus myth. The *means* suggested to him by his unknown predecessor are Laius's means: exposure to the elements. What if the Oedipus complex were a distorted version of the Laius complex? Rather than the representation of an infantile fantasy, the myth would then become a projection onto the child of a parental fantasy of infanticide. The oracle who warns Laius would thus be an externalization of a father's anxieties, an externalization that gives him the justification he needs to murder his own son. The attribution of evil intent to the child justifies evil intent on the part of the father. Tullio Hermil himself explains the underlying mechanism:

> Il piccolo fantasma perverso era una emanazione diretta del mio odio; aveva contro di me la stessa inimicizia che io avevo contro di lui; era un nemico, un avversario col quale stavo per impegnare la lotta. Egli era la mia vittima ed io era la sua. (*L'Innocente,* 540)

> [That perverse little phantom was a direct emanation of my hatred; it harbored the same hostility against me that I harbored against it; it was an enemy, an adversary with whom I was about to take up battle. He was my victim and I was his.]

Tullio is caught in a family romance in which, however, motives for murder exist on the part of the father as well as that of the son. His confession through denegation is impressively economical, for he thus commits fratricide, parricide, and infanticide in one condensed stroke. The mythological subtexts are too many, the variations on the family romance too obsessive, the rhetorical mechanisms too similar not to suspect that D'Annunzio here is discovering Freud's terrain before Freud has even set foot on it. D'Annunzio's rendering of the discourse of an *alienato* suggests the presence of unconscious mechanisms that limit and distort Hermil's true confession, mechanisms that, Freud will claim, are proper to oneiric discourse. The "true" confession lies elsewhere; another narrative lies "behind" that of the novel, recounting the tortuous paths taken by Hermil's sexuality and psychology. The logic is that which we have come to label Freudian, but its narrativization in D'Annunzio's text produces a kind of scrambling of the Freudian code. We might say, in fact, that *L'Innocente* is not a rereading but a prereading of the Freudian account of Oedipus.

"As you know," wrote Freud, "every discovery is made more than once and none is made all at once."[29] The suggested parallel between D'Annunzio and Freud is precisely that: the two contemporaries (Freud, seven years D'Annunzio's elder, died one year after the poet) explore similar problems, and though their modes of

29. Sigmund Freud, "The Sense of Symptoms," *Standard Edition,* 16:257.

analysis and conclusions may ultimately be dissimilar, both "discover" the unconscious. By way of Lombroso and the Lombrosian narrator of *L'Innocente,* D'Annunzio's meditation on the relationship of bodies to thought opens onto very non-Lombrosian conclusions, and his search for a language with which to describe "stati d'animo" leads him to a rhetoric of the unconscious. But this particular discovery is tied to a particular body—the upper-class male body; the rhetoric of sickness as applied to the upper-class female body is, as we shall see in the final chapter, quite a different matter.

[4] *Pandora's Box*

Transgressions

Neither Baudelairean nor Lombrosian, the rhetoric of sickness as applied to the upper-class female body might be labeled specifically D'Annunzian, for it constitutes the erotic discourse of the *Romanzi della Rosa*. Convalescence appears once again, and once again as the identity of the convalescent is altered, so too is the ideology thus embodied.

The sickness from which the upper-class female character convalesces is often of a specifically female sort, as Mario Praz has noted in *The Romantic Agony:*

> Both Tullio Hermil and Giorgio Aurispa have intercourse with women who are scarcely convalescent from diseases of the womb [malattie della matrice]. Elena gives herself to Sperelli when she is ill. In Ippolita Giorgio possesses an epileptic, and Paolo Tarsis, in Isabella Inghirami, a lunatic. Sterility also, a characteristic of D'Annunzio's women, acts as a sadistic stimulus. "She is sterile. Her womb is accursed. . . . The uselessness of her love seemed to him a *monstrous transgression* against the supreme law" (*Trionfo della morte,* p. 361). Giorgio Aurispa is especially attracted by the bodily defects of Ippolita: "The most vulgar features had an irritating attraction for him" (p. 360). Stelio Effrena is excited by the *faisandage* of la Foscarina. A

"transgression" from the normal, in fact, seems to be a *sine qua non* of D'Annunzio's love stories.[1]

Praz's reading of sickness and sterility in D'Annunzio's female characters well represents the *doxa* of D'Annunzian criticism: sterility renders the woman a perfect instrument of voluptuous pleasure, sickness renders her a ready-made victim of the male protagonist's sadistic impulses. This reading, it should be noted, is less an interpretation than a repetition of the texts themselves. Tullio Hermil makes no bones about "la tanto esecrata perversione sadica" ["the so often execrated sadistic perversion"], and it is the narrator of *Trionfo della morte* who explains that Ippolita's sterility makes her "un più prezioso strumento di voluttà" ["a more precious instrument of voluptuousness"].[2] Yet Praz's observation that a transgression of a norm is necessary to D'Annunzio's erotic discourse seems as unconfutable as it is generic. Indeed, though Praz seems to limit this characteristic of erotic discourse to decadent writers of the likes of D'Annunzio, Baudelaire, and Swinburne, Georges Bataille, in *L'histoire de l'érotisme*, expands it to eroticism in general:

> The history of eroticism is not at all that of sexual activity allowed within the limits defined by *infractions of rules*. It is always a matter of going beyond the admissible limits: there is nothing erotic in sexual play that resembles that of animals. And perhaps eroticism is relatively rare (it is difficult to determine on account of the small amount of certain information we have): it consists in the fact that some received forms of sexual excitment take place in such a way that they are no longer receivable. It is therefore a matter of passing from the licit to the prohibited. The sexual life of man arose from the accursed, *prohibited* domain, not from the licit domain.[3]

1. Mario Praz, *The Romantic Agony*, trans. Angus Davidson, with a foreword by Frank Kermode (1951; rpt. London: Oxford University Press, 1978), 267.

2. Gabriele D'Annunzio, *L'Innocente*, in *Prose di romanzi, Tutte le opere di Gabriele D'Annunzio*, ed. Egidio Bianchetti (Milan: Mondadori, 1955), 1:394; D'Annunzio, *Trionfo della morte*, in *Prose di romanzi*, 1:1033.

3. Georges Bataille, *L'histoire de l'érotisme*, in *Oeuvres complètes* (Paris: Gallimard, 1976), 8:108.

Without prohibitions and transgressions there can, for Bataille as well as for D'Annunzio, be no eroticism. That D'Annunzio's erotic discourse concurs with Bataille's analysis is perhaps less interesting than the specific nature of the prohibitions transgressed in D'Annunzio's *Romanzi della Rosa*. Why, we might ask, should sickness constitute a prohibition at all? Naturalistic explanations are rendered inadequate by the nature of the diseases involved. In the three novels in question those diseases are not (at least medically speaking) communicable ones but instead, as Praz has observed, "malattie della matrice" and epilepsy. In fact, both diseases are particularly suited to constitute prohibitions not because, naturalistically speaking, they inhibit the sexual act, but because they are both figured as sacred diseases. Vivifying etymological and mythological connections, D'Annunzio attributes vaguely diagnosed uterine dysfunction to the action of "il dèmone isterico," and Ippolita's epilepsy is most often referred to as "il male sacro." The transgression seems thus not of social or medical norms but of some other, "divine" law established by the text.

This rhetoric of sickness, which evokes both sacred and demonic, is the erotic discourse of the *Romanzi della Rosa*. Broadly speaking, there is a movement in the trilogy from an eroticization of female sickness in *Il piacere* to its total deeroticization in *Trionfo della morte*. The erotic effect of such illnesses upon the male protagonist undergoes an apparent cyclical evolution, tracing what Paolo Valesio has described as the ideological frame that shapes D'Annunzio's erotic politics in general: "The symbolic action of erotic relationships in D'Annunzio's novels follows, generally, a basic double movement: first a movement of triumphant assertion (conquest, enjoyment), soon followed by dissatisfaction, repentance, and a general flight away from the flesh and its 'pleasures.'"[4] This could stand as an accurate thematic description of the entire cycle of the *Romanzi della Rosa*, with *Il piacere* as the moment of conquest and enjoyment, *L'Innocente* as the moment of repentance, and *Trionfo della morte* as the moment of the flight from the flesh. The final "flight" of *Trionfo della morte*, however, marks the beginning of some other "phase" only in the sense that it leads to a "refinement"

4. Paolo Valesio, "The Lion and the Ass: The Case for D'Annunzio's Novels," *Yale Italian Studies* 1.1 (1977): 71.

of the preceding movement. D'Annunzio's experiment with physio-logical description seems to end with *Trionfo della morte*, not only because of his acquaintance with Nietzsche's philosophy, but be-cause his modern "romance of the rose" is already an unveiling that concludes that veils are necessary. In *Le vergini delle rocce* we no longer find an alternation between conquest and revulsion, nor do we find physiological descriptions of either male protagonist or female object of desire. The rhetorical strategy of *Le vergini delle rocce* is that of allegoresis, and the erotic discourse in that work, as well as in *La Gioconda* and *Il fuoco*, is essentially a fetishistic one that eroticizes "dismembered" objects—hair, voice, hands—and avoids any description of the "rose" itself.[5] We might therefore rewrite the "ideological frame" in less Christian terms (or at least as doubting Thomas rather than penitent sinner) as a moment of revelation followed by disbelief and, finally, disavowal, for an unveiling that concludes that veils are necessary is nothing other than the fetishist's disavowal.[6] In differing forms, the novels of the trilogy narrativize the logic of fetishism, and the "law" transgressed is the law that constitutes sexual difference.

The Hysterical Demon

Physiological description of specifically female ailments is lim-ited to several apparently isolated episodes in *Il piacere*. Sperelli lives in anticipation of conquest for the greater part of the novel, and moments of revelation are few. Those few moments coincide

5. For a discussion of allegoresis in *Le vergini delle rocce*, see Lucia Re, "Gabriele D'Annunzio's Novel *Le vergini delle rocce*: 'Una cosa naturale vista in un grande specchio,'" *Stanford Italian Review* 3 (Fall 1983): 241–71.

6. The Nietzschean ring to this formulation is intentional. See the Preface to *The Gay Science*, ed. and trans. Walter Kaufmann (1887; New York: Vintage Books, 1974), 38: "We no longer believe that truth remains truth when the veils are withdrawn." See Sarah Kofman's analysis of the relation between veils and fetishism in her chapter "Baubo: Perversion théologique et fétichisme," in *Nietzsche et la scène philosophique* (Paris: Union Générale d'Editions, 1979), as well as Derrida's discussion of truth and veils in *Spurs: Nietzsche's Styles/Eperons: Les styles de Nietzsche*, trans. Barbara Harlow (Chicago: University of Chicago Press, 1979).

with the appearance of a rhetoric of sickness and are the germ of the (repulsive) revelation that will become the dominant tone of *Trionfo della morte,* and of the fetishistic revelation manqué of *La Gioconda.*

As Praz has noted, Sperelli and Elena first consummate their flirtation in Elena's sickbed. The malady from which she suffers appears to be the "nevralgie della faccia" ["neuralgia of the face"] mentioned as an affliction to which Elena is prone. It remains unnamed in the scene and we learn only that "la signora soffriva molto e che non poteva veder nessuno" ["the lady suffered greatly and could not see anyone"].[7] Sperelli, however, an exception to this rule, is allowed to enter the sickroom. As he crosses the threshold, he is struck by an odor: "Ebbe, da prima, l'impressione d'un'aria assai calda, quasi soffocante; sentì nell'aria l'odore singolare del cloroformio" (*Il piacere,* 85) ["He had at first the impression of rather hot, almost stifling air; he smelled the singular odor of chloroform"]. The presence of chloroform in the sickroom might suggest that "vapors" or "female troubles" are being treated, though the pain from which Elena suffers is localized in the face: "Gli angoli esterni delle palpebre si restringevano per la contrazion dolorosa dei nervi infiammati" (*Il piacere,* 85) ["The outer corners of her eyelids were contracted by the pain of her inflamed nerves"].[8] But if the first mention of chloroform, as Sperelli enters the room, is an indicator of Elena's pain, the second, upon his exit, links the sickroom to pleasure, to an erotic effect upon Sperelli: "Gli persisteva nel senso l'odore di cloroformio, simile a un vapore di ebrezza" (*Il piacere,* 88) ["The odor of chloroform lingered in his senses, like an intoxicating vapor"]. This hint of an eroticization of sickness is not developed further in *Il piacere,* but remains a suggestion which will be taken up in *L'Innocente,* for one of the threads of continuity between the two novels can be traced from the sickbed seduction in *Il piacere* to Giuliana, who rarely leaves her sickbed in *L'Innocente.*

Giuliana is permanently convalescent in *L'Innocente;* the surgery

7. Gabriele D'Annunzio, *Il piacere,* in *Prose di romanzi,* 1:81.

8. Chloroform was available as a pain-killer, used in particular to ease the pains of childbirth, from 1847 on. Its growing use in obstetrics and gynecology was controversial in the latter half of the century, as Peter Gay documents in *Education of the Senses,* vol. 1 of *The Bourgeois Experience: Victoria to Freud* (New York: Oxford University Press, 1984), 226–33.

she undergoes in the *incipit* is followed by a long convalescence from which she emerges not healthy but pregnant. In her already weakened condition, that pregnancy becomes yet another illness that confines her to her bed until childbirth nearly causes her death. Giuliana manages to get out of bed only long enough to get into bed with Filippo Arborio. This eternally bedridden woman is a phenomenon of the nineteenth century well documented by social historians.[9] Giuliana might be said, in fact, to be a textbook case of female invalidism. As Barbara Ehrenreich and Deirdre English point out in their book on the sexual politics of sickness, "Not only were women seen as sickly—sickness was seen as feminine."[10] True to this ideologeme of the sick woman, Giuliana's invalidism, her languor and unearthly pallor render her all the more desirable. In *L'Innocente,* the femininity of sickness is overdetermined, for we find not merely a sick woman but a woman who suffers from "female troubles," from "malattie complicate della matrice e dell'ovaia" (*L'Innocente,* 378) ["complicated disease of the womb and of the ovaries"].

The female troubles that plague Sperelli are of a different sort. The scene of Sperelli's convalescence, from which Elena is necessarily excluded, terminates their affair. When Sperelli returns in book 3 to his life of pleasure, the valence carried by female pathology is no longer a positive one.

The dinner scene that opens book 3 marks Andrea's return to Roman high society and to the "perversion" that had preceded his short-lived conversion to art. This return to perversion is figured as a return of the physiology so carefully avoided in the scene of convalescence. The androgynous Maria, the ventriloquist's ideal, is supplanted by the hermaphroditic Bébé Silva, who becomes a caricature of both Maria and the feminized Sperelli:

9. See, for example, Elaine Showalter, *The Female Malady: Women, Madness, and English Culture, 1830–1890* (New York: Pantheon, 1985). For a discussion of the effect of this phenomenon on the woman writer, see Sandra M. Gilbert and Susan Gubar, *The Madwoman in the Attic: The Woman Writer and the Nineteenth-Century Literary Imagination* (New Haven: Yale University Press, 1979), in particular the chapter "Infection in the Sentence: The Woman Writer and the Anxiety of Authorship," 45–92.

10. Barbara Ehrenreich and Deirdre English, *Complaints and Disorders: The Sexual Politics of Sickness* (Old Westbury, N.Y.: Feminist Press, 1973), 22.

Ella somigliava un collegiale senza sesso, un piccolo ermafrodito vizioso: pallida, magra, con gli occhi avvivati dalla febbre
e dal carbone, con la bocca troppo rossa, con i capelli corti,
lanosi, un po' ricci, che le coprivano la testa a guisa d'un
caschetto d'*astrakan*. Teneva incastrata nell'occhiaia sinistra
una lente rotonda; portava un alto solino inamidato, la cravatta
bianca, il panciotto aperto, una giacca nera di taglio maschile,
una gardenia all'occhiello, affettando le maniere d'un *dandy*,
parlando con una voce rauca. E attirava, tentava, per quella
impronta di vizio, di depravazione, di mostruosità, ch'era nel
suo aspetto, nelle sue attitudini, nelle sue parole. (*Il piacere*,
253)

[She resembled a sexless schoolboy, a vice-ridden little hermaphrodite: pale, thin, her eyes brightened by fever and kohl,
her mouth too red. Her hair, short, woolly and slightly curled,
covered her head like an astrachan helmet. She held a round
lens tightly in her left eye. She wore a high starched collar,
a white necktie, an open waistcoat, a black jacket of a masculine
cut and a gardenia in her buttonhole. She affected the manners
of a dandy and spoke with a husky voice. And she enticed,
she tempted, precisely on account of that imprint of vice,
depravity, and monstrosity in her appearance, her attitudes,
and her words.]

Bébé Silva is a monstrosity precisely because she is a degraded
embodiment of the "ideal androgyne." Along with her fellow
demimondaines, she is the object in this episode of a facile misogyny
that insists on "la dolce ignoranza di quelle belle oche" (*Il piacere*,
251) ["the sweet ignorance of those pretty geese"]. The young men
are quite entertained by the women's inability to understand Latin
and by their lack of historical knowledge. The narrator cannot be
similarly faulted, as he demonstrates by reviving a topos as ancient
as the Egyptian papyruses:

Quel vino chiaro e brillante, che ha su le donne una virtù così
pronta e così strana, già incominciava ad eccitare variamente
i cervelli e le matrici di quelle quattro etàire ineguali, a
risvegliare e a stimolare in loro il piccolo dèmone isterico e a

farlo correre per tutti i loro nervi propagando la follia. Bébé
Silva gittava motti orribili, ridendo d'un riso soffocato e
convulso e quasi singhiozzante come quel d'una donna che sia
per morir di solletico. *(Il piacere, 255)*

[That light and sparkling wine which has such an immediate
and such a strange effect upon women had already begun to
excite, variously, the brains and wombs of those four unequal
hetairai, and to awaken and stimulate in them the little
hysterical demon and cause it to run through their nerves,
propagating madness. Bébé Silva tossed out horrible mottoes,
laughing a suffocated, convulsed, almost sobbing laugh like
that of a woman about to die from tickling.]

While the young men flaunt their knowledge of Latin, D'Annunzio
shows off his knowledge of Greek. As though to alert the reader
(whose Greek may be no better than Bébé Silva's Latin) that the
hysteria of which he speaks is Hippocratic rather than Freudian
(with an added touch from early Christian demonology), D'Annunzio prepares the ground by referring to the demimondaines, with
the Greek term for courtesan, *hetaira.* His use of *isterico* is thus
similarly Greek, referring specifically to the womb, *hystera.* D'Annunzio is both etymologically and medically exact in his revival of
the topos of the "wandering womb." Wine was, in fact, thought
to excite the uterine animal; in some cures wine was proscribed for
a year in order to halt the womb's peregrinations.[11] Bébé Silva's
"hysterical fit" is precisely and etymologically that: convulsions
resembling those of epilepsy and suffocation were the principal
symptoms of a wandering womb.[12]

11. This cure appears in Aulus Cornelius Celsus's treatise "On Diseases of
the Womb," where, according to Ilza Veith, "Celsus recommended that the
therapy be extended an entire year in order to avoid recurrence and that wine
be proscribed for the same length of time." Ilza Veith, *Hysteria: The History of
a Disease* (Chicago: University of Chicago Press, 1965), 21.
12. Veith summarizes the Hippocratic text *On the Diseases of Women* in her
history of hysteria: "The thinking ran that in such situations the uterus dries up
and loses weight and, in its search for moisture, rises toward the hypochondrium,
thus impeding the flow of breath which was supposed normally to descend into
the abdominal cavity. If the organ comes to rest in this position it causes
convulsions similar to those of epilepsy. If it mounts higher and attaches itself

One might object that this is merely an archaic description of woman's physiology and not a description of a disease. Yet pathology is inherent in this description, and woman's physiology appears to be inseparable from pathology. Once begun, this fall into physiology acquires a momentum of its own and carries the text toward an equally pathological, if not equally ancient, topos, that of the enchantress turned hag:

Bébé Silva fumava, beveva bicchierini di *vieux cognac* e diceva cose enormi, con una vivacità artifiziale. Ma aveva a quando a quando, momenti di stanchezza, di prostrazione, stranissimi, ne' quali pareva che qualche cosa le cadesse dal volto e che nella sua figura sfrontata e oscena entrasse non so qual piccola figura triste, miserabile, malata, pensierosa, più vecchia della vecchiezza d'una bertuccia tisica che si ritragga in fondo alla sua gabbia a tossire dopo aver fatto ridere la gente. (*Il piacere,* 257)

[Bébé Silva smoked, drank tiny glasses of *vieux cognac,* and said outrageous things with an artificial vivacity. But from time to time she had the strangest moments of fatigue, of prostration, in which it seemed as though something fell from her face and into her brazen and obscene figure entered I don't know what sad, wretched, sick, pensive little figure, older than the old age of a consumptive monkey that withdraws to the corner of its cage to cough after having made people laugh.]

This topos functions as a moment of revelation: a reality concealed by artifice is unveiled. But what is the nature of the reality so

to the heart the patient feels anxiety and oppression and begins to vomit. When it fastens itself to the liver the patient loses her voice and grits her teeth, and her complexion turns ashen. If the uterus lodges in the loins, the woman feels a hard ball, or lump, in her side. But when it mounts as high as the head, it causes pains around the eyes and the nose, the head feels heavy, and drowsiness and lethargy set in. Beyond these specific symptoms, the movement of the womb generally produces palpitations and excessive perspiration and convulsions similar to those observed in epilepsy" (10–11). Hysteria was also thought of as suffocation of the womb, "suffocation of the Mother."

revealed, and why is it figured as female? Canto 7 of Ariosto's
Orlando furioso, in which the enchantress Alcina's magic is undone
by Melissa, is undoubtedly an intertext to the D'Annunzian description and may begin to provide an answer:

> Pallido, crespo e macilente avea
> Alcina il viso, il crin raro e canuto,
> sua statura a sei palmi non giungea:
> ogni dente di bocca era caduto;
> chè più d'Ecuba e più de la Cumea,
> ed avea più d'ogni altra mai vivuto.
> Ma sì l'arti usa al nostro tempo ignote,
> che bella e giovanetta parer puote.
>
> Giovane e bella si fa con arte,
> sì che molti ingannò come Ruggiero;
> ma l'annel venne a interpretar le carte,
> che già molti anni avean celato il vero.

[She was whey-faced, wrinkled, and hollow-cheeked; her hair
was white and sparse; she was not four feet high; the last tooth
had dropped out of her jaw; she had lived longer than anyone
on earth, longer than Hecuba or the Cumaean Sibyl. But she
made such use of arts unknown in our day that she could pass
for young and fair. Young and fair she made herself by artifice,
and deceived many as she deceived Ruggiero. But now, with
the ring, he could read the card aright and see the truth which
for so many years had been kept hidden.][13]

The reality revealed by this commonplace is usually represented by
an old, shrunken, toothless woman who is the bearer of disease or
vermin. D'Annunzio eliminates toothlessness; Ariosto, disease.
Machiavelli, in a 1509 letter to Luigi Guicciardini, eliminated
neither and minced no words in elaborating upon the topos. The
woman in question is not first described as beautiful and in the

---

13. Ludovico Ariosto, *Orlando furioso,* ed. Lanfranco Caretti (Milan: Ricciardi, 1954), 7.73.1–74.4; the translation is that of Guido Waldman (London:
Oxford University Press, 1974), 69.

flower of youth, though Machiavelli had clearly expected that she would be comely:

Venendomi pure voglia di vedere questa mercatanzia, tolsi un tizzone di fuoco d'un focolare, che v'era, ed accesi una lucerna, che vi era sopra. Nè prima el lume fu appreso, che 'l lume fu per cascarmi di mano. Omè fu' per cadere in terra morto, tanto era brutta quella femina. E' se le vedeva prima un ciuffo di capelli fra bianchi e neri, cioè canuticci, e, benchè l'avessi el cocuzzolo del capo calvo, per la cui calvizie a lo scoperto si vedeva passeggiare qualche pidocchio, nondimeno pochi capelli e rari le aggiugnevano con le barbe loro infino in su le ciglia. E nel mezzo della testa, piccola e grinzosa, aveva una margine di fuoco, chè la pareva bolata a la colonna di Mercato. In ogni punto delle ciglia di verso li occhi aveva un mazzetto di peli pieni di lendine; li occhi li aveva uno più basso ed uno alto; ed uno era maggiore che l'altro; piene le lagrimatoie di cispe ed e' nipitelli dipellicciati. El naso li era confitto sotto la testa, arricciato in su, e l'una delle nari tagliata, piena di mocci. La bocca somigliava quella di Lorenzo de' Medici, ma era torta da un lato, e da quella n'usciva un poco di bava, chè, per non aver denti, non poteva ritener le sciliva. Nel labbro di sopra aveva la barba lunghetta, ma rara. El mento aveva lungo, aguzzato, torto un poco in su; dal quale pendeva un poco di pelle, che le aggiungeva infino a la facella della gola. Stando attonito a mirar questo mostro, tutto smarrito, di che lei accortasi, volle dire: —Che avete voi messere? —Ma non lo disse, perchè era scilinguata. E, come prima aperse la bocca, n'uscì un fiato sì puzzolente, che, trovandosi offesi da questa peste due porte di dua sdegnosissimi sensi, li occhi e il naso, e messi a tale sdegno, che lo stomaco, per non poter sopportare tale offesa, tutto si commosse. E, commosso, oprò sì che io le rece' addossi; e così, pagata di quella moneta che la meritava, mi partii.

[I had the urge to see my merchandise and I took a brand from the fireplace near me and lit a lamp that was above it; and hardly was it lit when the light almost dropped from my hand. My God! The woman was so ugly that I almost dropped dead. The first thing I noticed was a tuft of hair, half white and half black, and although the top of her head was bald, which allowed you to observe a number of lice taking a stroll, nevertheless a few hairs mingled with the whiskers that grew around her face; and on top of her small, wrinkled head there was a scar-burn which made her look as if she had been branded at the market; her eyebrows were full of nits; one eye looked down, the other up, and one was larger than the other. Her tear ducts were full of mucus and her eyelashes plucked; her nose was twisted into a funny shape, the nostrils were full of snot, and one of them was half cut off; her mouth looked like Lorenzo de' Medici's, but it was twisted on one side and drooled a bit since she had no teeth to keep the saliva in her mouth; her upper lip was covered with a thin but rather long moustache; her chin was long and sharp, pointed up, and from it hung a bit of skin that dangled to her Adam's apple. As I stood there, amazed at this monster, she noticed my surprise and tried to say: "What is the trouble, sir?"; but she could not, since she was a stutterer; and as she opened her mouth there came from it such such a stinking breath that my eyes and my nose, the two gateways of the two most outraged senses, found themselves offended by this pestilence; this was such a shock to my stomach that, not being able to bear it, it heaved so much that I vomited all over her. And so, having paid her in the way she deserved, I left.][14]

Machiavelli's description is certainly more Folenghian than Ariostean, but the basic outlines are the same. The old woman's hair is thin and whitish; her mouth, toothless. Virilization is part of uglification, just as it is an element of Bébé Silva's monstrosity; facial hair and (Machiavelli couldn't resist a stab at the Medici) a mouth that resembles Lorenzo's render her even more repulsive. It is striking that the description pans no lower than the woman's

---

14. Niccolò Machiavelli, "Spectabili viro L. Guicciardini in Mantova tanquam fratri carissimo," in *Lettere,* ed. Guiseppe Lesca (Florence: Rinascimento del Libro, 1929), 26–27, translated as "To Luigi Guicciardini in Mantua," in *The Portable Machiavelli,* ed. and trans. Peter Bondanella and Mark Musa (New York: Penguin, 1979), 59–60.

throat; all emphasis is placed upon facial dissymmetry and, more important, upon various excretions from her facial orifices: "cispe," "mocci," "bava" ["mucus," "snot," "drool"]. Machiavelli's "due porte di dua sdegnosissimi sensi" ["two doors of two outraged senses"] are especially offended by the stinking breath that issues from this stuttering woman's mouth. These last details—stuttering and foul odor—send us to yet another such revelatory moment in which, however, a different "porta" is in question: the episode of "la femmina balba" in *Purgatorio* 19. Here there is a double movement from initial ugliness and deformation—

> mi venne in sogno una femmina balba
> ne li occhi guercia, e sovra i piè distorta,
> con le man monche, e di colore scialba.

[There came to me in a dream a woman, stammering, with eyes asquint and crooked on her feet, with maimed hands, and of sallow hue.]

to enchantment, as she is transformed into a siren—

> Poi ch'ell'avea 'l parlare così disciolto
> cominciava a cantar sì che con pena
> da lei avrei mio intento rivolto.

> "Io son", cantava, "io son dolce serena
> che 'marinari in mezzo al mar dismago;
> tanto son di piacer a sentir piena!"

[When she had her speech thus unloosed, she began to sing so that it would have been hard for me to turn my attention from her. "I am," she sang, "I am the sweet Siren who leads mariners astray in mid-sea, so full am I of pleasantness to hear."]

and then to the moment of disenchantment, revelation, and revulsion—

L'altra prendea e dinanzi apria
fendendo i drappi, e mostravami 'l ventre;
quel mi svegliò col puzzo che n'uscia.

[He seized the other and laid her bare in front, rending her
garments and showing me her belly: this waked me with the
stench that issued therefrom.][15]

Unveiling is here made literal ("fendendo i drappi") and the truth
so revealed is a literalization of the "bocca sdentata" [toothless
mouth] of the preceding descriptions. Emphasis on the mouth,
breath, and facial excretions in Machiavelli's letter appears as a
displacement upward of a horror that regards what D'Annunzio in
Cento e cento e cento pagine calls "l'autre bouche" ["the other
mouth"].[16] Such displacement facilitates a transfer between a "bocca
sdentata" and a "vagina dentata." It is interesting, then, that
D'Annunzio only includes a portion of the topos, omitting the
toothless mouth. Such reticence is little more than a touch of
delicacy in terms of our analysis of a text; by employing such a
classic topos, he evokes the entire landscape that topos describes.

The topos of the enchantress turned hag is often read, by both
critics and the writers themselves, as an attack not on women but
on artifice in general and rhetoric in particular. As a figure for
hermeneutics itself, it may be read as enacting the discovery of
essence that lies beneath appearance, truth beneath falsehood, reality beneath fiction, plain speech beneath cosmetic rhetoric. Indeed,
as we have seen, Nietzsche uses this very topos in order to overturn
it, in order to critique the hermeneutic model that would find an
essence beneath appearance. These are, of course, valid interpretations. Yet they discard the literal in order to concentrate on the
figural and thus do not ask why woman is favored as the vehicle of
the metaphor. What interests me here, however, is not only the

15. The edition used is Dante Alighieri, *La commedia secondo l'antica vulgata*,
ed. Giorgio Petrocchi, 4 vols. (Milan: Mondadori, 1966–67), *Purgatorio*, 19.7–
9, 16–21, 31–33; the translation is that of Charles Singleton, *The Divine Comedy*,
with a commentary by Singleton (Princeton: Princeton University Press, 1973).

16. Gabriele D'Annunzio, *Cento e cento e cento pagine del libro segreto di Gabriele
D'Annunzio tentato di morire*, in *Prose di ricerca, Tutte le opere di Gabriele D'Annunzio*,
ed. Egidio Bianchetti (Milan: Mondadori, 1968), 2:754.

tenor but also the vehicle, for in *Il piacere* we are dealing with a rhetoric of eros. The truth hidden by artifice is a double one: the truth concealed by Sperelli's rhetoric is a "truth" about woman's body, a truth that, as Machiavelli demonstrates, may be difficult to stomach.

When this topos appears in a discourse on eros, the figurative meaning sends us back to the literal meaning. Because it functions as an attack on artifice, the "truth" put forth disturbs the erotic effect of such discourse. The revelation unveils the "falsity" of Sperelli's rhetoric of uniqueness, for it uncovers a truth about woman's body, a "repulsive" common denominator shared by all women. Neither Elena nor Maria may now be *L'Unica,* nor can Sperelli be *L'Unico:*

> L'impurità, che *allora* la fiamma alata dell'anima velava d'un velo sacro e circondava d'un mistero quasi divino, appariva ora senza il velo, senza il mistero della fiamma, come una lascivia interamente carnale, come una libidine bassa. Ed egli sentiva che quel suo ardore non era l'Amore e che non aveva più nulla di comune con l'Amore. Non era l'Amore. Ella gli aveva gridato: —Soffriresti tu di spartire con altri il mio corpo? —Ebbene, sì, egli l'avrebbe sofferto. (*Il piacere,* 261)

> [The impurity that the winged flame of the soul had *then* veiled with a sacred veil and surrounded with an almost divine mystery, now appeared without the veil, without the mystery of the flame, as a wholly carnal lasciviousness, as a low lust. And he felt that this ardor of his was not Love, and no longer had anything in common with Love. It was not Love. She had cried: "Could you bear to share my body with others?" Well, yes, he would bear it.]

As the veils of Sperelli's rhetoric are rent, so too are the veils of Elena's charms; for the first time, she is described dispassionately:

> La sua facoltà precipua, il suo *asse* intellettuale, per dir così, era l'imaginazione; un'imaginazione romantica, nudrita di letture diverse, direttamente dipendente dalla matrice, continuamente stimolata dall'isterismo. Possedendo una certa in-

telligenza, essendo stata educata nel lusso d'una casa romana
principesca, in quel lusso papale fatto di arte e di storia, ella
erasi velata d'una vaga incipriatura estetica....Ella copriva
di fiamme eteree i bisogni erotici della sua carne e sapeva
transformare in alto sentimento un basso appetito. (*Il piacere,*
268)

[Her principal faculty, her intellectual *axis,* so to speak, was
imagination; a romantic imagination, nourished with wide
reading, directly dependent upon her womb, constantly stim-
ulated by hysteria. Possessed of a certain intelligence and
brought up in the luxury of a princely Roman house, in that
papal luxury made of art and history, she had veiled herself
with a vague aesthetic cosmetic. . . . She covered the erotic
needs of her flesh with ethereal flames and knew how to
transform a low appetite into a noble sentiment.]

Under the *fiamme eteree* we find another *etàira.* Elena's veils are
classier than Bébé Silva's, but like that of Bébé Silva and her
companions, Elena's "incipriature estetica" is washed away in order
to reveal both a psychological and a physiological truth about
woman: her psychology is indistinguishable from her physiology,
"direttamente dipendente dalla matrice." But if her psychology is
determined by her physiology, and physiology (and physiological
description) are, as D'Annunzio seems to suggest in these passages,
inherently antierotic, then another solution must be found in order
to perpetuate an eroticized erotic discourse. Sperelli discovers his
solution by transforming the principle of interchangeability, only
just discovered by drawing back the veils, into a new veil. He can
eroticize his discourse and intercourse by superimposing an image
of another woman upon the woman to whom he makes love:

Quella voce! Com'erano strani nella voce di Donna Maria gli
accenti d'Elena! —Gli balenò un pensiero folle. —Quella
voce poteva esser per lui l'elemento d'un'opera d'imaginazione:
in virtù d'una tale affinità egli poteva fondere le due bellezze
per possederne una terza imaginaria, più complessa, più per-
fetta, *più vera* perchè ideale. (*Il piacere,* 294)

[That voice! How strange were Elena's tones in the voice of Donna Maria! A mad thought flashed before him. That voice could be the element of a work of the imagination for him: by virtue of such an affinity, he could combine their two beauties in order to possess a third, imaginary beauty, more complex, more perfect, *more true* because ideal.]

Though the result obtained appears truer, the strategy employed is still veiling. An image of one woman masks the physical reality of another; the technique is so effective that he takes the veil for reality when he calls Maria, Elena.

Prometheus and Pandora

"Egli non potrebbe credere al fallo di Giuliana." Were we to translate D'Annunzio's *L'Innocente,* this phrase might give us pause: He could not believe in Giuliana's offense? He could not believe in Giuliana's defect? He could not believe in Giuliana's . . . phallus? The pause might last but a moment, for surely we would cede to contextual pressure and choose the first of these versions: Tullio Hermil's brother, Federico, could not believe in Giuliana's error, in her offence, in her infidelity. We might rest assured that this, after all, is what the text *means.* But if we allow homonymy to speak, we find that the text asks questions of a different order: Could he believe in Giuliana's lack? Could he believe in Giuliana's phallus? Homonymy rends the text of *L'Innocente,* for *fallo* in Italian may mean all these things: error, mistake, or equivocation; a physical or spiritual defect, failing, or imperfection; a sin or offence; the emblem of the virile member or the organ itself.[17] This particular case of homonymy opens dizzying possibilities for psychoanalytic discourse, for that which the woman lacks, *il fallo,* might be referred to by that very same term, *fallo* (her imperfection, her defect), and the recognition of this *fallo* (her failing, her defect) is itself the source of error and equivocation, yet another *fallo.*

17. Paolo Valesio first brought this homonym to my attention in a lecture "The Psychoanalysis of the Sword," Symposium on Sex and Language, New York City, 1 May 1981.

Psychoanalysis would no longer be able to tell this particular story of haves and have-nots.

These possibilities, brought into view by the problem of translation, are not simply the result of a play upon the semantic richness and etymological difference of a homonym. *Fallo* is, in the text of *L'Innocente*, what Michael Riffaterre has called a dual sign, "an equivocal word situated at the point where two sequences of semantic or formal associations intersect. . . . These parallels meet, in defiance of geometric law, only because the dual sign properly placed in one of the two sequences would have been just as at home in the other."[18] Privileged as dual signs are cases of homophony and, in particular, of homonymy. The dual sign may at first appear to be a pun, especially when, like paronomasia, it relies upon homophony. But while a pun's pungency is also based on homophony, its immediate context *insists* upon the transfer from homophony to synonymy. The pun in pungency, for example, is drawn out by its proximity to "pun"; the worse the pun (and "pungency" is a bad one), the more attention must be drawn to it by its context. A dual sign, instead, belongs simultaneously to two different texts: what Riffaterre has termed the mimetic, syntagmatic text, and the semiotic, paradigmatic text. Its "context-bound" syntagmatic meaning may well be "incompatible with the context-free paradigmatic significance." The dual appropriateness of the dual sign will be brought forth not by its immediate context, as in the case of a pun, but by an act of retroactive reading: "retroactive reading thus appears to be the method for decoding dual signs: first, because the sign refers to a paradigm, and a paradigm can be recognized

18. Michael Riffaterre, *The Semiotics of Poetry* (Bloomington: Indiana University Press, 1978), 86. One of Riffaterre's examples concerns the word *oublie* (a kind of wafer sold in the street) that, in a passage taken from Chateaubriand, appears in a funereal context such that its homophone, *oubli*, emerges in an "other text": "What is happening here is the overdetermination of the word *oubli(e)*, doubly appropriate: it is generated by an associative chain of street-scene words, but also by a chain of mourning and death words" (88). Cynthia Chase analyzes another occurrence of this same dual sign, *oublie/oubli*, in Rousseau's *Neuvième promenade*, in connection with Baudelaire's "abusive translation" of this sign into yet another dual sign, *diligence*, in "La morale du joujou." See her "Paragon, Parergon: Baudelaire Translates Rousseau," in *Decomposing Figures: Rhetorical Readings in the Romantic Tradition* (Baltimore: Johns Hopkins University Press, 1986), 196–208.

only after it has been sufficiently developed in space so that certain constants can be perceived; second, because any stumbling block sends the reader scurrying back for a clue, back being the only place to go; third, because the correction made backwards via the proximate homologue creates the ghost or parallel text wherein the dual sign's second (or syntactically unacceptable) semantic allegiance can be vindicated."[19] Such a "ghost text" is precisely what we find in L'Innocente, for while the immediate, mimetic context forces us to read the syntactically acceptable "offence," the paradigmatic context allows us to read "phallus/failing." The ghost text to which these "secondary" associations belong is L'Innocente as an interpretation of the myth of Oedipus. The "secondary" fallo— the failing, the phallus—is found at a crucial interpretive moment in this scrambled oedipal narrative.

As we have seen, a chiastic reversal takes place between the incipit and the second section, or second beginning. In the second section, Giuliana's infidelity is revealed and the narrative focuses not on Tullio's but on Giuliana's fallo and on the resultant pregnancy that becomes her "morbo." Giuliana's fallo, her sin, is inseparable from the fallo, the phallus:

> Orbene, ella si dà a un uomo, commette il suo primo fallo,
> e rimane incinta, ignobilmente, con la facilità di quelle fem
> mine calde che i villani sforzano dietro le siepi, su l'erba in
> tempo di foia. (L'Innocente, 517)

> [So, she gives herself to a man, commits her first error (fallo)
> and gets pregnant, ignobly, with the ease of those hot females
> whom peasants rape behind bushes on the grass when they
> are in heat.]

This transfer of characteristics is, mimetically speaking, a transference of guilt: Tullio relinquishes his "imagine fallica" by projecting it onto Giuliana.

But Giuliana already had a fallo of a different sort. In the incipit, she too was afflicted by a "morbo ignoto," her vaguely diagnosed uterine dysfunction:

19. Riffaterre, 91.

Seppi, dopo, che già da alcuni mesi la travagliavano malattie complicate della matrice e dell'ovaia, quelle terribili malattie nascoste che turbano in una donna tutte le funzioni della vita. (*L'Innocente, 378*)

[I later discovered that already for several months complicated diseases of the womb and the ovaries had tormented her, those terrible hidden diseases that disturb all the functions of life in woman.]

These terrifying hidden ills conveniently enough allow Tullio to avoid all erotic contact with Giuliana, and the discovery of them arrives almost as a wish fulfillment. One might expect these hidden ills to act as an antiaphrodisiac, to cause anxiety or disgust in Tullio. This is, in fact, the interpretation that is placed in the mouth of Giuliana:

— Di' —mi chiese un giorno, con la bocca amara—se tu ci pensi, non hai ribrezzo di me? Ah, che brutta cosa! E fece un atto di disgusto su sè medesima; e s'accigliò, e si ammutolì. (*L'Innocente, 379*)

["Tell me," she asked one day, her mouth full of bitterness, "if you think of it, are you repulsed by me? Oh what an ugly thing!" And she made a gesture of repugnance at herself, frowned and fell silent.

Her physician concurs and institutionalizes this presumed disgust by insisting that all erotic contact be avoided, thereby suggesting a purely naturalistic interpretation of both her malady and the prohibition it installs:

Il dottore, col quale volli avere un colloquio, mi fece intendere che per un lungo periodo io doveva rinunziare a qualunque contatto con la malata, anche alla più lieve delle carezze; e mi dichiarò che un nuovo parto avrebbe potuto esserle fatale. (*L'Innocente, 378*)

[The doctor with whom I insisted on speaking gave me to

understand that I must renounce all contact, even the slightest of caresses, with the sick woman for some time. And he stated that another pregnancy might be fatal.]

Tullio himself, however, adds a prohibition of a different sort when he imagines the gynecological operation she must undergo. His description cuts to the heart of the matter, to the real nature of both terror and taboo, for this is no ordinary operation:

Ah, così mi parve, morente mi parve, quella mattina, quando i dottori l'addormentavano col cloroformio ed ella, sentendosi sprofondare nell'insensibilità della morte, due o tre volte tentò di alzare le braccia verso di me, tentò di chiamarmi. Io uscii dalla stanza, sconvolto; e intravidi i ferri chirurgici, una specie di cucchiaio tagliente, e la garza e il cotone e il ghiaccio e le altre cose preparate su un tavolo. Due lunghe ore, interminabili ore, aspettai, esacerbando la mia sofferenza con l'eccesso delle imaginazioni. E una disperata pietà strinse le mie viscere d'uomo, per quella creatura che i ferri del chirurgo violavano non soltanto nella carne miserabile ma nell'intimo dell'anima, nel sentimento più delicato che una donna possa custodire: — una pietà per quella e per le altre, agitate da aspirazioni indefinite verso le idealità dell'amore, illuse dal sogno capzioso di cui il desiderio maschile le avvolge, smanianti d'inalzarsi, e così deboli, così malsane, così imperfette, uguagliate alle femmine brute dalle leggi inabolibili della Natura; che impone a loro il diritto della specie, sforza le loro matrici, le travaglia di morbi orrendi, le lascia esposte a tutte le degenerazioni. E in quella e nelle altre, rabbrividendo per ogni fibra, io vidi allora, con una lucidità spaventevole, vidi la piaga originale, la turpe ferita sempre aperta "che sanguina e che pute." (L'Innocente, 383)

[Dying! Oh, that is how she appeared to me that morning when the doctors put her to sleep with chloroform, and she, feeling herself sink into the insensibility of death, tried two or three times to lift her arms toward me, she tried to call me. I left the room, upset. And I glimpsed the surgical instruments, a sort of sharp spoon, and the gauze and the cotton and the ice and all the other things ready on a table. Two long, interminable hours I waited, exacerbating my suffering with an excess of fantasies. And in my male viscera I felt a pang of desperate pity for that creature whom the surgical instruments violated not only in her wretched flesh but in the recesses of her soul, in the most delicate sentiment that a woman can defend—a pity for her and for the others, tormented by indefinite aspirations toward the idealities of love, deluded by the captious dream with which masculine desire surrounds them, yearning to raise themselves up, and so weak, so sickly, so imperfect, made equal to the females of the brutes by the unabolishable laws of Nature, which imposes upon them the law of the species, strains their wombs, torments them with horrible maladies, leaves them exposed to all kinds of degeneration. And in that one, and in the others, shivering in every fiber, I saw then, with a frightening lucidity, I saw the original wound, the foul wound, always open, "that bleeds and stinks."]

The description marks above all a moment of revelation: what is hidden about the nature of her disease is revealed. The sight itself belongs to that "other" text within the text of *L'Innocente,* and is marked by the contrast between the (mimetic) "intravidi" and the (oneiric) "vidi...vidi." What Tullio sees is an interpretation of a perception: as he imagines the surgical operation, it becomes a repetition of a primal "operation" at the hand of nature: woman's castration. The foul wound that bleeds and stinks represents Giuliana's, and woman's ("in quella e nelle altre"), first *fallo,* her lack of a phallus. The sight of woman's wound is the sight of the Medusa, but though the narrator professes pity for these poor creatures, a pity that provokes a sympathetic reaction in his "viscere d'uomo," a fear that a similar fate might befall him remains implicit.[20] He is not frozen in fearful recognition but instead feels the stirrings of

---

20. For Freud, of course, the terror of Medusa is "a terror of castration that is linked to the sight of something," and that "something" is the woman's *lack* of a penis. See his "Medusa's Head," *The Standard Edition of the Complete Psychological Works of Sigmund Freud,* trans. James Strachey (1961; rpt. London: Hogarth Press, 1978), 18:273–74.

a desire to repeat the scene of this operation, to reproduce its effects. The "memory" that, in the narrator's flow of associations, precedes and evokes Tullio's vision of the operation represents a desire to reeffect her castration in their intercourse:

> La violenza del desiderio sarebbe in me attenuata dalla paura di farle male, di strapparle un grido di dolore. —Dopo tanto! —E i nostri esseri, all'urto di una sensazione divina e terribile, non provata nè imaginata mai, si struggerebbero. Ed ella, dopo, mi parebbe quasi morente, con la faccia tutta molle di pianto, pallida come il suo guanciale. Ah, così mi parve, morente mi parve, quella mattina. (L'Innocente, 383)

> [The violence of my desire would be attenuated by the fear of hurting her, of drawing a cry of pain from her. "After so much!" And our beings, under the shock of a divine and terrible sensation, never before experienced or imagined, would melt. And afterwards, she would seem almost as though she were dying, with her face soft with tears and pale as her pillow. Ah, that is how she seemed, as though she were dying, that morning.]

The results of their lovemaking should mime the results of her operation. D'Annunzio did not, of course, invent the figuration of orgasm as death, but the immediate association of her "wound" and their lovemaking suggests a specific means of "dying." When this imagined scene moves from the conditional into the indicative, and Giuliana and Tullio rediscover passion at Villalilla, Giuliana's cries of "sono morta" ["I am dead"] act as a seductive prelude to their union.

There is, however, more to Hermil's fascination with Giuliana's "loss" than the desire for her repeated castration. Hermil, whose rhetoric is the accumulation of ever new sensations, suspects that Giuliana may have gained something else by having, as it were, nothing to lose:

> La malattia, forse, aveva aumentata, esasperata quella sensibi-lità. Ed io pensai, curioso e perverso, che avrei veduto la debole vita della convalescente ardere e struggersi sotto la mia

carezza; e pensai che la voluttà avrebbe avuto quasi un sapore d'incesto. "Se ella ne morisse?" pensai. Certe parole del chirurgo mi tornavano alla memoria, sinistre. E per quella crudeltà che è in fondo a tutti gli uomini sensuali, il pericolo non mi spaventò ma mi attrasse.(*L'Innocente*, 393)

[The illness had perhaps increased and exasperated her sensitivity. And curious and perverse, I thought that I would have seen the feeble life of the convalescent burn and melt beneath my caress. And I thought that the voluptuous pleasure would almost have a taste of incest. "If she were to die of it?" I thought. The surgeon's words returned to me, sinister. And because of that cruelty that lies at the base of all sensual men, the danger did not frighten me, but attracted me.]

Hermil's voluntary admission of sadistic impulses and incestuous yearnings might provide an adequate explanation of the aphrodisiac effect of Giuliana's illness and wound were it not that in the 1903 *Laus vitae* the wound "che sanguina e che pute" reappears. The body upon which it is inflicted is, however, no longer female:

> Gli Efimeri onorano il càuto
> Ribelle, oblioso del tuo
> Ordine puro che solo
> generò l'Universo!
> La piaga che sanguina e che pute
> nell'egro fegato, sotto
> il rostro del vùlture adunco,
> ai lamentevoli figli
> del Rimorso e della Paura
> la piaga la piaga stridente
> ahi più venerabile sembra
> che la tua solitaria fronte
> ove balzò l'unica nata
> Pallade Atena dagli occhi
> chiari vergine prode
> artefice meditabonda
> patrona dei vertici forti
> nemica del cieco tumulto

> lucida regolatrice
> del combattimento ordinato
> che reca al sicuro trionfo![21]

[The ephemeral ones worship the cautious Rebel, forgetful of your pure Order that alone generated the Universe! The wound that bleeds and stinks in the sick liver, under the hooked beak of the vulture, oh the wound, the strident wound seems more venerable to the lamentable sons of Remorse and of Fear than does your solitary brow whence bounded forth your only born, Pallas Athena of the bright eyes, the intrepid virgin, meditative artifex, patron of strong summits, enemy of blind tumult, lucid regulatrix of ordered combat that leads to certain triumph!]

The wound here described is that of cunning Prometheus, punished by Zeus for having stolen fire and given it to men. His, too, is a "piaga originale," for the Prometheus myth is also a myth of the origin of the "damnable race of women."[22] The binding of Prometheus was only a part of his punishment; the other half was

---

21. Gabriele D'Annunzio, *Maia,* in *Versi d'amore e di gloria, Tutte le opere di Gabriele D'Annunzio,* ed. Egidio Bianchetti (Milan: Mondadori, 1950), 2:84.

22. Hesiod recounts Prometheus's story in both the *Theogony* and *The Works and Days,* placing little emphasis on the wound and accentuating instead the creation of Pandora as Prometheus's principal punishment. In the *Theogony,* Athena appears as accomplice to Zeus in the creation of Pandora: "In return for the theft of fire he instantly produced a curse to plague mankind. At the orders of the son of Cronus, the famous lame smith-god shaped some clay in the image of a tender girl. The bright-eyed goddess Athena dressed and decked her in silvery clothes. A marvelous embroidered veil fell from her head and was held in her hands. Round her head the goddess tied a golden diadem on which the smith-god himself had exercised his skill, to please his father Zeus. When Zeus had completed this beautiful curse to go with the blessing of fire, he displayed the girl in an assembly of gods and men, all decked out in the finery supplied by the bright-eyed daughter of the lord of hosts. Gods and men were speechless when they saw how deadly and irresistible was the trick with which Zeus was going to catch mankind. This was the origin of the damnable race of women— a plague which men must live with." Hesiod, *Theogony,* ed. and trans. Norman O. Brown (Indianapolis: Bobbs-Merrill, 1953), 69–70.

the gift of Pandora to men, a curse to accompany the blessing of fire. The image of Prometheus as midwife to the birth of women is reinforced by variations that figure him as instrumental to the birth of Athena; he is said to have struck Zeus's brow with an axe (thus causing another wound) at the propitious moment.[23] D'Annunzio's omission of Pandora, of the creation of woman, is thus only apparent, for the abrupt comparison to Zeus's parturition of Athena serves the same symbolic function as would a mention of Pandora. Prometheus's wound is indissolubly linked with the origin of women; D'Annunzio's equation of Prometheus's and woman's wound suggests a reading of the Prometheus and Pandora myths such that Prometheus himself becomes woman, becomes Pandora. The symbolic, displaced castration of the myth is returned to its original site: it is Prometheus's wound that releases sickness and travail upon the human race:

> L'odor della carne corrotta
> del sudore anèlo,
> della febbre, dell'agonia,
> della putredine ha vinto
> l'ambrosia della tua chioma
> su' tuoi grandi pensieri
> ondeggiante, o Generatore
> incorruttibile.
> (*Maia*, 84–85)

[The odor of corrupted flesh, of panting sweat, of fever and agony and putridity has conquered the ambrosia of your mane,

23. Apollodorus relates Zeus's "conception" and parturition of Athena: "From fear of that [that Metis should bear a son who would be lord of heaven] Zeus swallowed her. And when the time came for the birth to take place, Prometheus or, as others say, Hephaestus, smote the head of Zeus with an axe, and Athena, fully armed, leaped up from the top of his head at the river Triton." Apollodorus, *The Library*, trans. Sir James George Frazer (London: Heinemann, 1921), 25. For a survey of the many versions of the Prometheus myth, from Hesiod to Gide, see Jacqueline Duchemin, *Prométhée: Histoire du mythe, de ses origines orientales à ses incarnations modernes* (Paris: Société d'édition "Les belles lettres," 1974).

undulating above your great thoughts, O incorruptible Generator.]

In the oldest version of the myth, Hesiod's *Works and Days,* this is precisely what Pandora releases from the vase she bears as a gift from Zeus to men.[24] The description of Giuliana's wound in *L'Innocente* is faithful to this version, for her "piaga originale" is the matrix of "morbi orrendi" and "tutte le degenerazioni."

If Prometheus and Pandora are condensed into one figure, then we might say that Giuliana too is both a Prometheus and a Pandora. She is marked by a Promethean wound and bears the ills that plague mankind. The introduction of the myth of Prometheus suggests that access to knowledge is gained only at the price of woman's wound. That wound and its attendant illnesses are the price Prometheus must pay for his knowledge of the arts and of fire.[25] It is as though woman herself were a figure for transgression and the knowledge gained thereby. But she possesses yet another of Prometheus's characteristics: though she is the bringer of degeneration, she also has, in her "wounded" organ, a capacity for continual regeneration. Just as Prometheus's liver grows back proportionately as it is eaten by the eagle, so do Giuliana's wounded

24. See Hesiod, *The Works and Days,* trans. Richmond Lattimore (Ann Arbor: University of Michigan Press, 1978), lines 90–102. The episode of the jar does not appear in the *Theogony.* In *Pandora's Box: The Changing Aspects of a Mythical Symbol* (New York: Pantheon, 1956), Dora and Erwin Panofsky trace to Erasmus the origin of Pandora's "box" as a mistranslation of the Greek *pithos.* It seems that only the Italian "vaso di Pandora" remains faithful to the original: "The only exception is, characteristically, Italy, less deeply committed to Erasmus than the transalpine world. Here the vernacular adhered, and adheres to this day, to 'vaso di Pandora,' and only the Latin-writing humanists—unless they were conscientious or pedantic enough to retain the orthodox 'dolium'— inclined to yield to the Erasmian fashion, at least to the extent of reducing the size of the vessel to that of a 'vasculum'" (19). Apart from Italy's relationship to Erasmus, however, there are lowlier reasons for such philological accuracy. If the vernacular continues to adhere to *vaso,* it is probably because *la scatola di Pandora* would have rather different connotations: *le scatole* refers to testicles.

25. According to Plato's *Protagoras,* Prometheus stole wisdom in the arts together with fire but not civic wisdom, which was in the possession of Zeus. See Plato, *Laches, Protagoras, Meno, Euthydemus,* trans. W. R. M. Lamb (London: William Heinemann, 1972), 320c–322d.

organs "grow back" by producing a child. This connection between women's reproductive organs and Prometheus's wounded organ does not go unexplored in classical mythology. The story of Tityus "repeats" Prometheus's story, making explicit that which is already implicit in the myth, for Tityus's organ grew again with each new cycle of the moon; the regeneration of his organ thus follows the model of the menses.[26] It is this regenerative ability, and the pregnancy that results from it, which is the source of Tullio's distress in the novel and, on at least one occasion, quite explicitly the source of his passion for Giuliana. Soon after learning of her pregnancy, Tullio makes violent love to her, hoping thereby to dislodge the developing fetus. It is as though he played the part of the eagle, reopening the "original wound." The desire to repeat her castration is grounded in a phantasy of continual regeneration of woman's *fallo:* woman is not castrated once and for all but, like Prometheus, wounded again and again. Hermil is caught in a reenactment, a repetition of the moment of discovery: again and again, the woman must regain her *fallo* in order to lose it; again and again, Hermil must castrate the woman in order to save his own *fallo.*

At this point, the dual sign *fallo* points us beyond the story of haves and have-nots to a different psychoanalytic tale of haves-who-have-not: fetishism. In his desire to repeat the moment of discovery, Hermil can be likened to Freud's fetishists who retain their belief that women have a phallus at the same time as they give up that belief. The fetish is, for Freud, the sign of the presence of something (specifically, of the mother's penis) and at the same time of its absence. The "subtlest" fetish accomplishes precisely this: Freud cites the case of a man whose fetish was a *Schamgürtel,* a "suspensory belt" that could be worn as either undergarment or bathing drawers and whose wearer could as easily have a male member as not have it, as easily be a have as a have-not. It thus suspended the decision between present and absent phallus, and the fetishist could simultaneously deny and accept the "fact" of woman's defect, of woman's

26. As punishment for having attempted to rape Leto, Tityus was stretched upon the ground "while two vultures or snakes ate his heart or liver, which grew again with each new cycle of the moon." See Edward Tripp, *The Meridian Handbook of Classical Mythology* (New York: New American Library, 1970), 580.

phallus, of woman's *fallo:* "Analysis showed that it signified that women were castrated, and that they were not castrated; and it also allowed of the hypothesis that men were castrated, for all these possibilities could equally well be concealed under the belt."[27] Hermil's phantasy of Promethean regeneration narrativizes the fetishist's divided attitude by turning the fetishist's simultaneous disavowal and affirmation of castration into sequential and infinitely repeatable moments.

But the similarities between fetishism and the text of *L'Innocente* are not limited to a thematic level, to a discussion of the mental process named by fetishism. They touch upon the process of signification as well: the dual sign *fallo* is itself a fetish on the level of language. Not only is *fallo* the sign of something's presence and of its absence, but like Freud's suspensory belt, it allows defect and phallus to coexist. *Fallo* is, linguistically, the perfect fetish, for when the word itself is read retroactively, it is equally at home in two texts: in the mimetic text of perception ("there is nothing there, no penis"), and the semiotic text of interpretation ("there must have been one, but now it is castrated"). At the same time it performs a metalinguistic function, for it *names itself* as equivocation, as *fallo*. Neither dual sign nor fetish (when understood as "suspensory belt") can be considered either a metaphor (as is assumed in common usage of the term *fetish*) or a metonymy (as in the cases Freud describes, where the last thing seen before the moment of discovery—shoes, pubic hair—then becomes the fetish) but both are, as Riffaterre says of the dual sign, "at once catachresis and the right word."[28] If catachresis is the "abuse of figure," a "metaphor" that does not substitute for a literal term (as in the "leg of a table" or the "eye of the storm"), then we might consider the woman's *fallo* to be a catachresis. *Fallo is* the woman's phallus: the penis she never had and yet was castrated, just as the "leg of the table" is the leg it never had and yet is lame, a "wooden leg." That is, just as there is no literal, proper way to say "leg" of the table, there is no literal way to say "penis of the woman"; and just as, in giving the table a leg, language mutilates it and ourselves, so in giving the woman a penis, woman—and man—is wounded,

27. See Freud, "Fetishism," *Standard Edition,* 21:156.
28. Riffaterre, 92.

castrated.[29] The table indeed has "something" that we call a leg (indeed, it is said to have a "head" as well), but naming it "leg" has amputated that leg from the body it does not have; woman has "something" yet that something is neither the presence nor the absence of a penis/phallus, but the equivocation named by *fallo*. Thus it is not so much the character Tullio who is fetishistic as the text itself, which creates such an undecidable fetish.

As in the case of the Oedipus myth, D'Annunzio's reading of castration is a scrambling of the Freudian code. It does not, I think, move outside of the possibilities foreseen in Freud's texts. Indeed, I have implied that the child is, in some sense, the woman's phallus just as Freud will claim that the woman's desire to have a child is a desire for the organ she lacks. What D'Annunzio's text suggests, however, is that the child-as-phallus provides a motive for infanticide on the part of the father.

But the story does not end here, for it is not only Giuliana who becomes both Prometheus and Pandora. The Prometheus-Pandora story is a powerful myth of transgression and its consequences,

29. See Andrzej Warminski's analysis of catachresis as self-mutilation in *Readings in Interpretation: Hölderlin, Hegel, Heidegger* (Minneapolis: University of Minnesota Press, 1987), liii–lxi. In *Stanze: La parola e il fantasma nella cultura occidentale* (Turin: Einaudi, 1977), Giorgio Agamben sees in the fetishist's *Verleugnung* the possibility of a model of signification no longer "under the sign of Oedipus," that is to say, no longer a hermeneutic scheme according to which metaphor (and meaning) is constituted by the substitution and exchange of improper and proper terms: "What the *proper/improper* schema prevents us from seeing is that in reality nothing is substituted for anything in metaphor, because there is no proper term that the metaphorical term is called to substitute: only our ancient oedipal prejudice—that is, an *a posteriori* interpretive schema—makes us see a substitution where there is only a dislocation within a single process of meaning [un unico significare]. . . . One can say, rather, that *Verleugnung* offers a model for the interpretation of metaphor that escapes from the traditional reduction of the problem, and in the light of that model *metaphor becomes in the realm of language that which the fetish is in the realm of things*. As in *Verleugnung* there is not in fact a 'transfer' ['trasporto'] from a proper or improper meaning" (177–78). At precisely this moment, when Agamben would like to propose a new linguistic model ("in the realm of language"), he has recourse to visual representations, to emblems and caricature, as examples and thus begs the question of language itself by amalgamating it to other semiotic systems. Catachresis might have served him better, since it is precisely in catachresis that the "proper/improper" schema is jettisoned.

and thus it might easily be recuperated in the commonplace that D'Annunzio's erotic discourse is transgressive. The truth of that commonplace is irrefutable insofar as any erotic discourse is bound to set up prohibitions in order to transgress them. The question we must ask, then, is what law is being transgressed in D'Annunzio's text? Hermil's open admissions of incestuous desires, sadistic impulses, actual infanticide, and infidelity now appear to be misleading clues that tell us there is indeed a transgression, while throwing up a smoke screen that obscures the true nature of the transgression involved. Naturalistic explanations of woman's "sickness" as prohibition are also inadequate, for that disease is the contagion of castration.

The conflation of Prometheus and Pandora becomes, in fact, a powerful metaphor of the writer for whom eviration represents a desirable state. In both *L'Innocente* and *Il piacere,* scenes of the male protagonist's convalescence are preceded by scenes of dueling and therefore by the threat of a wound. Those convalescences are figured as conversions to aesthetic and moral values and are the scene of the protagonist's feminization. In *Il piacere* a rediscovery of the arts is specifically linked to Sperelli's wound; Sperelli is wounded in a duel at the close of book 1 and it is from this wound that he ostensibly convalesces. Hermil is not physically wounded, but instead meets his rival at a fencing club, assesses Arborio's skill as a fencer, and learns that he is to duel the following day. The narrative structure is the same in both cases: a scene of dueling ends the opening section and prepares the ground for the protagonist's feminization and convalescence. Hermil's feminization occurs by less direct means when, in the two succeeding chapters he takes on Giuliana's role and qualities as a "spiritual" convalescent. But Tullio, too, is metaphorically wounded, for his conversion to goodness is contingent upon his separation from Teresa Raffo, the "imagine fallica" that had led him astray. In order to gain pardon, he must expiate his sin: "Lo so, lo so; tutti i miei dolori non valgono forse il tuo dolore, non valgono le tue lagrime. Io non ho espiato il mio fallo, e non sono degno d'essere perdonato" (*L'Innocente,* 449) ["I know, I know; all my sufferings are not equal to your suffering, are not equal to your tears. I have not expiated my sin/phallus [*fallo*] and I am not worthy of being forgiven"]. Once again, homonymy rends the text, for Tullio must expiate both sin and phallus.

The feminization undergone by both male protagonists remains an indirect eviration rather than castration. Physiological description, assiduously avoided, reappears instead as a description of organic disturbance not in the "viscere d'uomo" but in "la matrice femminile." The most female of ills is chosen to figure the most male of fears; Giuliana's sickness, her vaguely diagnosed uterine dysfunction, thus appears as a displacement of Tullio's "castration."

Hermil professes to desire sadistically the castration of the other, yet his own feminization suggests that he might also identify with this "castrated" being, as he does during what is presented as Giuliana's second surgical operation, childbirth: "Soffrivo anch'io uno strazio fisico, simile forse a quello d'un'amputazione mal praticata e lentissima. Gli urli della partoriente mi giungevano a traverso l'uscio" (*L'Innocente*, 578) ["I, too, suffered physical torture, perhaps similar to that of a clumsy and very slow amputation. The screams of the woman giving birth reached me from across the threshold"]. This comparison of childbirth to an amputation undergone by the protagonist points once again to the transference of a fantasy of castration onto Giuliana. Giuliana is more desirable following this "amputation," just as she had become desirable after her first operation. Giuliana becomes the castrated, wounded being Tullio desires, and desires to be; the feminized Tullio's desire for her is thus almost a desire for his own castration in her. Here lies Tullio's true transgression, for he too would become both Prometheus and Pandora.

A Sacred Disease

Trionfo della morte continues and enlarges upon themes from *Il piacere* and *L'Innocente*. Sperelli's preoccupation with finding "L'Unica" becomes Giorgio Aurispa's obsession, while Tullio Hermil's obsession with paternity becomes Aurispa's dread and desire. The rhetoric of female sickness embodies both concerns in this, the final novel of the trilogy, where the dominant moment is that of flight from the flesh and revulsion at the moment of revelation.

Aurispa's goal is total possession of his lover: "C'è su la terra una sola ebrezza durevole; la *sicurtà* nel possesso di un'altra creatura, la sicurtà assoluta incrollabile. Io cerco questa ebrezza" (*Trionfo,* 796) ["There is only one lasting intoxication on earth: *certainty* in the possession of another creature, absolute, unshakable certainty"]. The major obstacle to such possession is not the uncertainty of the present or future, but the irrevocability of the past. The first two sections, "Il passato" and "La casa paterna," represent this obstacle and establish the themes of priority and fatherhood which will dominate in the novel. Those themes, according to Harold Bloom, are the preoccupations of the poet. In his analysis of the relationship between poet and muse, Bloom observes that the desire for the one-and-only woman and the poet's attitude toward his muse appear to be similarly motivated:

> If he himself is not to be victimized, then the strong poet must "rescue" the beloved Muse from his precursors. Of course, he "overestimates" the Muse, seeing her as unique and irreplaceable, for how else can he be assured that *he* is unique and irreplaceable? Freud dryly remarks that "the pressing desire in the unconscious for some irreplaceable thing often resolves itself into an endless series in actuality," a pattern particularly prevalent in the love life of most poets, or perhaps of all post-Romantic men and women cursed with strong imagination.[30]

The desire to be unique raises the problem of priority, for possession of the muse—or of mortal women—can only be complete if the poet is her "first": "If this is to serve as a model for the family romance between poets, it needs to be transformed, so as to place the emphasis less upon phallic fatherhood, and more upon *priority,* for the commodity in which poets deal, their authority, their property, turns upon priority."[31]

These two aspects of the family romance, phallic fatherhood and priority, are precisely Aurispa's concerns. Yet he can achieve neither, and Ippolita's illnesses come to represent the impossibility

30. Harold Bloom, *The Anxiety of Influence: A Theory of Poetry* (1973; rpt. London: Oxford University Press, 1981), 63.

31. Ibid., 61.

of possession and priority in erotic matters. Ippolita is afflicted with both "il dèmone isterico" ["the hysterical demon"] and "il male sacro" ["the sacred ill"], diseases that appear as the continuing presence of the past in her body, and which figure her prior possession by others.

Like Elena and Giuliana, Ippolita is governed by "il dèmone isterico." But here uterine ills take on yet another meaning, for Ippolita's "malattia della matrice" appears as as the record of her previous sexual experience. Her prior possesion is recorded in a peculiarly female sort of memory:

> "Una tale donna" egli pensava "è stata d'altri prima che mia! Ha giaciuto con un altro uomo; ha dormito con un altro uomo nel medesimo letto, sul medesimo guanciale. In tutte le donne è singolarmente viva una specie di memoria fisica, la memoria delle sensazioni." (*Trionfo,* 830)

> ["A woman like this," he thought, "has belonged to others before she was mine! She has lain with another man; she has slept with another man in the same bed, on the same pillow. In all women a sort of physical memory, the memory of sensations, is singularly alive."]

Woman's physiological memory manifests itself as disease, for the origin of her malady is traced to her marriage and sexual initiation:

> Ippolita era andata a nozze nella primavera avanti quella dell'amore. Dopo alcune settimane le era incominciata la malattia della matrice, lenta e crudele, che, riducendola in fondo a un letto, l'aveva tenuta per molti giorni sospesa tra la vita e la morte. Ma la malattia per fortuna l'aveva salvata da qualunque altro contatto odioso con l'uomo che s'era impadronito di lei, come d'una preda inerte. (*Trionfo,* 830)

> [Ippolita had been married the spring before their love. After several months, the disease of the womb had begun, slow and cruel. It had confined her to her bed and for many days held her suspended between life and death. But fortunately the

disease saved her from any further contact with the man who
had taken possession of her, as of an inert prey.]

If her ailment is a welcome obstacle to further relations with her
husband, it is also an obstacle to her *jouissance* with Aurispa.
Though Ippolita claims to be a sort of emotional virgin, not having
yet experienced the "voluttà dell'amore," her "isteralgia" appears
to be inseparable from the memory of her loss of virginity:

> Ma a poco a poco, di giorno in giorno, una sensibilità latente
> aveva incominciato a risvegliarsi nelle fibre di lei intorpidite
> dal morbo, ancóra addolorate dagli spasimi dell'isteralgia,
> ancóra forse dominate da un istinto ostile contro un atto già
> parso odioso nelle orribili notti nuziali. (*Trionfo,* 831)

> [But little by little, day by day, a latent sensitivity had begun
> to awaken in her fibers numbed by the malady and perhaps
> still in pain from the spasms of hysteralgia, still dominated
> by an instinct hostile to an act that had previously, in those
> horrible nuptial nights, seemed odious to her.]

It is as though Ippolita's physiological memory were indelibly
implanted in her body. The memory seems to have been obliterated
when, following her introduction to the "voluttà dell'amore," Ippolita appears to have undergone a transformation and become
"another" woman. Yet respite is temporary, for that physiological
memory contains not only her sexual initiation but her social origins
as well. Her beauty is contaminated by both sexuality and her petit
bourgeois roots:

> Non erano belli i piedi nudi ch'ella a volta a volta scaldava su
> la ghiaia e rinfrescava nell'acqua; erano anzi difformati nelle
> dita, plebei, senz'alcuna finezza; avevano l'impronta manifesta
> della bassa stirpe. Egli li guardava intentamente; non guardava
> se non quelli, con uno straordinario acume di percezione e di
> esame, come se le particolarità della forma dovessero rivelargli
> un segreto. E pensava: "Quante cose fermentano nel suo
> sangue! Tutti gli istinti ereditarii della sua razza sono in lei,

indistruttibili, pronti a svilupparsi ed ad insorgere contro qualunque constrizione." (*Trionfo*, 941)

[Her bare feet, which by turns she warmed on the gravel and cooled in the water, were not beautiful; rather, the toes were deformed and plebeian, without any refinement. They bore the clear imprint of low origins. He stared at them intently; he watched only them, with an extraordinary sharpness of perception and of examination, as though the peculiarities of their form would reveal a secret to him. And he thought: "How many things ferment in her blood! All the hereditary instincts of her race are in her, indestructible, ready to develop and rise up against every restraint."]

Such a biological memory is precisely what Aurispa fears, not so much in Ippolita as in himself, for it is his own heredity that is perceived as inscribed in Ippolita's body. It is this genetic fatalism, rather than merely Ippolita's sterility, which leads him to renounce the perpetuation of both his own life and life in general. Death triumphs in this novel because the flight from the flesh is total; Aurispa flees not only from the "flesh" of the sexual act but from his own flesh and blood.

Though Aurispa's insistence upon Ippolita's sterility suggests that he wishes to become a father, his descriptions of his own flesh and blood point to a more fundamental problem: how to become a father without becoming his own father. Only Aurispa's mother is exempt from the "germi ereditati dal padre" ["germs inherited from the father"]; his Aunt Gioconda with her typhoid breath, his sister Cristina and her sickly child, his brother Diego, and even his uncle Demetrio, dead by his own hand to avoid a worse fate— all seem to be contaminated by a hereditary fault:

Il suo pensiero, la sua attenzione andarono al padre, con un passaggio spontaneo. Diego era il vero erede di quell'uomo.

Pingue, sanguigno, possente, quell'uomo pareva emanare dalle sue membra un perpetuo calore di vitalità carnale. Le mascelle assai grosse; la bocca tumida e imperiosa, piena d'un soffio veemente; gli occhi torbidi e un po' biechi; il naso grande, palpitante, sparso di rossore; tutte le linee del volto portavano l'impronta della violenza e della durezza. Ogni gesto, ogni attitudine aveva l'impeto d'uno sforzo, come se la musculatura di quel gran corpo fosse in lotta continua con l'adipe ingombrante. La carne, la carne, questa cosa bruta, piena di vene, di nervi, di tendini, di glandule, d'ossa, piena di istinti e di bisogni; la carne che suda e che dà lezzo; la carne che si difforma, che s'ammala, che si piaga, che si copre di calli, di grinze, di pustole, di porri, di peli; questa cosa bruta, la carne prosperava in quell'uomo con una specie di impudenza, dando al delicato vicino una impressione quasi di ribrezzo. "Non era, non era così, dieci, quindici anni fa; non era così" pensava Giorgio. "Io ricordo bene che non era. Sembra che questa espansione d'una brutalità latente, insospettata, si sia compiuta in lui a poco a poco. Io, io sono il figliuolo di quest'uomo!" (*Trionfo,* 737)

[His thought and attention shifted to his father, in a spontaneous transition. Diego was truly that man's heir.

Fat, sanguine, powerful, that man seemed to exude from his members a perpetual warmth of carnal vitality. His jaws were heavy, his mouth tumid and imperious, full of a vehement breath, his eyes were turbid and sinister. His nose was large, palpitating, reddish; all the lines of his face bore the imprint of violence and toughness. Every gesture and attitude had the impetus of an effort, as if the musculature of that large body were locked in a continual struggle with its encumbrance of fat. The flesh, the flesh, this brute thing full of veins, nerves, tendons, glands, bones, full of instincts and needs, the flesh that sweats and stinks, the flesh that deforms and sickens and is wounded and covered with callouses, with wrinkles and pustules and warts and hairs, this brute thing flesh prospered in that man with a sort of impudence and gave an impression of revulsion to his refined neighbor. "No, he wasn't like this ten, fifteen years ago, he wasn't like this," thought Giorgio. "I remember well that he was not like this. It seems that this expansion of latent and unsuspected brutality has occurred little by little. And I, I am this man's son!"]

This vision of the father's flesh as the flourishing of disease is later magnified into the sanctuary scene, in which all imaginable illnesses and deformations of humankind are presented not as a projection of the father but as Ippolita's dream, as the unleashing of Pandora's box. As the transposition from the father to Ippolita suggests, this vision deeroticizes the flesh of the sexual act and motivates the most radical and irreparable unveiling of the *Romanzi della Rosa:*

> "Ah la solitudine, la libertà, l'amore senza vicinanza, l'amore per le donne morte o inaccessibili!" La presenza d'Ippolita gli impediva qualunque oblio; gli richiamava sempre l'imagine del congiungimento bestiale, della copula operata con gli organi escrementizii, dell'atto spasmodico sterile e triste ch'era omai divenuto l'unica manifestazione del loro amore. (*Trionfo,* 983)

> ["Ah solitude, freedom, love without closeness, love for dead or inaccessible women!" The presence of Ippolita obstructed forgetfulness; it always recalled the image of bestial conjunction, of the copula accomplished with the excremental organs, of the spasmodic, sterile, and sad act that had become the only manifestation of their love.]

Once the topos of "inter urinas et faeces nascimur" has been evoked ("gli organi escrementizii"), there is little salvation possible for an erotic discourse that speaks of the female body as the source of eroticism.

Yet even if Aurispa's genes were clean and Ippolita had come to him a virgin, Aurispa's desire for total possession could never be satisfied. Ippolita is afflicted by a sacred disease, epilepsy:

> Un terribile male, già da lei sofferto nell'infanzia, un male nervoso che aveva le forme dell'epilessia, era di nuovo apparso. Le lettere, con la data di agosto, ne parlavano. "Tu non imaginerai giammai lo sbigottimento ch'io ho nello spirito. La mia tortura maggiore è questa implacabile lucidezza della visione fantastica. Io *ti vedo* contorcerti, nell'accesso; *io vedo* i tuoi lineamenti scomporsi e illividirsi, i tuoi occhi volgersi disperatamente sotto le palpebre rosse di pianto... Io *vedo*

tutta la terribilità del male, come s'io ti fossi vicino..." (*Tri-onfo*, 710)

[A terrible ailment, which she had already suffered as a child, a nervous ailment that took the form of epilepsy, had appeared again. His letters, dated in August, spoke of it. "You can never imagine the fear that I have in my soul. My greatest torment is this implacable lucidity of imaginative vision. I *see* you writhing during the attack; I *see* your face become distorted and livid, your eyes roll desperately beneath their lids, red from crying... I *see* all the horror of your illness as though I were near to you..."]

The voyeuristic emphasis in this passage suggests that her convulsions are a parody of her ecstasy in love. And yet though this first mention of her disease appears to eroticize it, her epilepsy acquires quite different connotations after the sanctuary scene. In the tale of "La vergine Anna" epilepsy was never referred to as "il male sacro," but here D'Annunzio quite explicitly indicates that Ippolita suffers from a sacred ailment. At the end of the sanctuary scene, Aurispa is tormented by the recent vision of an epileptic, a vision he cannot separate from Ippolita:

Appariva e spariva il fantasma, quasi fosse il sogno della dormente, esternato e reso visibile. "S'ella si risvegliasse e in lei il male sacro?" pensava Giorgio, con un brivido intimo. "L'imagine che si forma nel mio cervello m'è forse trasmessa da lei." (*Trionfo*, 918)

[The phantasm appeared and disappeared, as though it were the dream of the sleeper, externalized and made visible. "If she should awaken and, with her, the sacred disease?" thought Giorgio, with an inner shiver. "This image that takes shape in my brain has perhaps been transmitted from her to me."]

As sacred (and demonic), epilepsy is a disease of possession, and so appears to figure the impossibility of any true priority, any total possession. The woman is already possessed, already of another. The attribution of epilepsy to Ippolita is a recognition of the insurmountable obstacles to the possession of the beloved; so it is that the novel must end with a murder-suicide, as Aurispa pushes and then accompanies Ippolita over a cliff. The solution the novel offers to the problem of priority is culmination: the decadent lover, like the decadent writer, chooses to be the end of a line rather than accept the impossibility of priority.

A Memorial to Medusa

> Bellezza medusèa, la bellezza dei romantici intrisa di pena, di corruzione, e di morte. La ritroveremo alla fine del secolo quando la vedremo illuminarsi del sorriso della Gioconda. (Mario Praz)

The final unveiling of *Trionfo della morte* puts an end to the rhetoric of physiological sickness which characterizes D'Annunzio's early prose works. Thereafter it will be the fetishist's disavowal that will prevail, and erotic discourse in his later works will elaborate upon the fetishistic strategy of *L'Innocente.* Though a full exploration of his later works lies beyond the scope—and intent— of this book, a final example of such a strategy will illuminate not only D'Annunzio's "evolution" but the consequences of the decadent's occupation of the woman's body.

As we have seen, fetishism names not simply an obsession with certain objects (as assumed in common parlance) but a particular logic that allows contradictory beliefs—affirmation and disavowal of castration—to coexist.[32] The sign of both presence and absence, the Freudian fetish may, in the patient's experience, be determined

32. As referring to a mode of signification, the term *fetishism* has been applied to situations that may or may not refer to castration. Giorgio Agamben, for example, argues that the Marxian "fetishism of commodities" is based on a similar logic: "And just as the fetishist never succeeds in completely possessing his fetish, because it is the sign of two contradictory realities, so the owner of a commodity can never enjoy it simultaneously as use-value and as exchange-value" (45). Derrida's "generalized fetishism" would include Hegelian *Aufhebung* and the "virgin mother" of Christianity. See Jacques Derrida, *Glas* (Paris: Galilée, 1974), and Gayatri Spivak's discussion of *Glas* in "Displacement and the Discourse of Woman," *Displacement: Derrida and After,* ed. Mark Krupnick (Bloomington: Indiana University Press, 1983), 169–95.

by metonymy, the last thing seen before the moment of "revelation" being a likely choice. But what happens when the fetish enters the literary text? Something that might be considered a fetish from a thematic point of view—a collection of cut-off braids, an obsession with feet—might not enter the economy of the text in the sense outlined here. Giorgio Agamben has suggested, in response to this problem, that a particular rhetorical figure, synecdoche, might be said to participate in the logic of fetishism:

> It is curious to observe how a mental process of a fetishistic sort is implicit in one of the tropes common to poetic language: synecdoche (and also in its close relative [nella sua parente prossima], metonymy). To the substitution of part for whole that it effects (or of an object contiguous to another) corresponds the substitution of a part of the body (or of a related object) to the complete sexual partner in fetishism. That this is not simply a superficial analogy is borne out by the fact that metonymic substitution does not exhaust itself in the pure and simple surrogation of one term for another; the substituted term is instead at once negated and evoked by its substitute in a procedure whose ambiguity closely recalls Freudian *Verleugnung*.[33]

Agamben's suggestion that synecdoche at once evokes and negates the "whole" for which it stands, that the presence of the "part" is the sign of the absence of the whole, is tantalizing but perhaps too totalizing. Are all synecdoches then fetishistic? Would a thematic obsession with feet or a collection of braids then necessarily hint at a fetishistic logic at the same time as it appeared in the text as a synecdoche for the whole, the body, of which it is a part?

In traditional rhetoric, of course, synecdoche names the figure in which the part stands for the whole (*pars pro toto,* or vice versa, *totum pro parte*), the part *refers* to the whole. In the case of fetishism, however, the status of the "whole" to which the "part" refers must be taken into consideration. When we say "all hands on deck," the hands stand for sailors in a way different from the way in which the fetish stands "for" the woman's (and ultimately the mother's)

33. Agamben, 40.

penis. In his extension of the notion of fetishism, Agamben seems to "forget" castration: the fetish comes to substitute the "partner sessuale completo," rather than the "woman's penis," and femininity is displaced instead onto metomymy, "sua parente prossima." The logic of fetishism thus becomes simply a way of "having one's cake and eating it too," of having the thing and its negation. But there is no "cake" to be had: the fetish itself does not stand *for* the woman's penis, does not *refer* to it, but rather stands in "its" place of absence just as a catachresis stands in the place of something for which there is no "proper" term. As Sarah Kofman reminds us, there is no "thing" to which the fetish refers:

> The mother's penis, the "thing itself," is always already a fetish invented by the child, a *belief* implying at once denial and affirmation of castration. There was never a "thing itself," but only ersatz, a sham, a prosthesis, an originary supplementarity as the panicked reaction of infantile narcissism. Adult fetishism is a repetition of this spontaneous infantile fetishism and is not a substitute for the "thing itself" or for truth; as substitute for the phantasmal penis of the mother, it always already implies the play of supplementary difference in the "thing itself."[34]

Thus if synecdoche is to be privileged as the trope of fetishism, it must be a synecdoche that cannot be made to refer to a "whole," to the thing itself, but only to other synecdoches, *pars pro parte.* It must, in other words, be a *catachrestic* synecdoche that puts "something" in the place of "nothing."[35]

Now, of all the "parts" that litter D'Annunzio's texts, none is more pervasive and eroticized (or more subject to a description as

34. Sarah Kofman, "Ça cloche," in *Lectures de Derrida* (Paris: Galilée, 1984), 136–37.

35. That the relation of part to whole is put into question by the castration complex is confirmed by Jean Laplanche, in *Problématiques II: Castration/Symbolisations* (Paris: Presses Universitaires de France, 1980): "One may then ask: in this severance that is castration, what is severed from what? By this I mean: if one cuts between the penis and the individual, which is the principal and which is the accessory? . . . Where is the subject in castration? . . . On the side of the castrated body, or rather on the side of that which is cut, the penis?" (25).

fetish in common parlance) than the hand.[36] Whiter than white, smoother than marble, the hand seems to stand for the woman. These hands would be just another exhibit in D'Annunzio's collection of precious objects and bric-a-brac were it not that this particular synecdoche is the basis for a narrative of mutilation in the drama *La Gioconda*. This narrative, in which synecdoche appears *as* mutilation, as catachrestic synecdoche, participates in and constructs the logic of fetishism.

The plot seems rather banal at first: a sculptor, convalescent after a suicide attempt, is still torn between his faithful, loving wife and a femme fatale, "La Gioconda." The choice between two women is an ethical choice between a life in art, "fuori delle leggi e fuori dei diritti umani" ["outside of laws and outside of human rights"], and a life of "domestic virtues." The two women confront each other. The desperate wife resorts to a lie, and tells the femme fatale that her husband no longer wishes to see her. Beside herself, the rival attempts to destroy the wondrously beautiful statue she had inspired. The wife attempts to save the statue, which, in its fall, severs her hands. She interprets her amputation as punishment for her falsehood; the husband returns to art and the femme fatale while the wife remains husbandless and handless. And banal it would remain—yet another fin-de-siècle variation on the immunity of aesthetics to ethics, framed by a mannered elaboration of Walter Pater's celebration of Da Vinci's enigmatic portrait—had the play ended here.[37] But the drama continues with a fourth act in which neither sculptor nor muse is present; there is only the amputee, and the scene of a child's discovery that her mother has no hands.

36. See for example Glauco Viazzi's catalogue of D'Annunzian hands in "Di alcune funzioni segniche e corrispondenze nelle *Vergini delle rocce*," *ES: Materiali per il '900* (June–August 1980): 29. Viazzi's notion of fetishism is precisely of the "common parlance" variety, and he does not include Silvia Settala's severed hands in his collection.

37. Pater's influential essay "Leonardo da Vinci" first appeared in the *Fortnightly Review* (November 1869). See Walter Pater, *The Renaissance*, ed. Donald L. Hill (Berkeley: University of California Press, 1980), 77–101. The prominence given the hands sculpted by Verrocchio in D'Annunzio's play can be read as homage to the prominence granted Verrocchio's sketch in Pater's essay. See Praz, *Romantic Agony*, for a survey of variations on the theme of La Gioconda.

It is above all this "excessive" fourth act that sends us back to reread the play as a mise-en-scène of the fetishist's *Verleugnung*.

This (almost comical) tragedy is about nothing if not hands and the rule of catachrestic synecdoche. Dedicated to Eleonora Duse "dalle belle mani" ["of the beautiful hands"], the play is somewhat mechanical in its composition, as though an assignment had been given a precocious schoolboy to write a theme on "hands." The mechanicity could be described in various ways: as the mechanicity of the writer's hand, as the mechanicity of the hand of destiny, as the mechanicity of catachrestic synecdoche that must continually refer only to other synecdoches. Set in a room that seems "ordinato dalle mani di una Grazia pensierosa" ["ordered by the hands of a pensive Grace"],[38] the tragedy of Lucio Settala, the sculptor who has "nelle sue mani una vita di fiamma" ["a life of flame in his hands"], and Silvia Settala, whose "care, care mani, coraggiose e belle . . . sono d'una straordinaria bellezza" ["dear, dear hands, courageous and beautiful . . . are of extraordinary beauty"] unfolds. Lucio participates in the now-familiar narrative of convalescence: his attempt to take his life by his own hand ("Con la mano medesima che aveva impresso della creta il segno di vita, con la mano medesima egli strinse l'arma e la rivolse contro il suo cuore" [309] ["With the very hand that had imprinted the sign of life in clay, with that very hand he had held the weapon and turned it against his heart"]) left him wounded, and his convalescence has taken on the appearance of a conversion. He appears reborn, childlike ("Sembra ch'egli rinasca. Dianzi aveva gli occhi d'un bambino" [233] ["He seems to be reborn. Just now he had the eyes of a child"]), and converted from the life of aesthetics to that of ethics. He receives his new life from the hands of his wife: "Io benedico la sera e l'ora che mi portarono moribondo in questa casa del tuo martirio e della tua fede per ricevere un'altra volta dalle tue mani— da queste divine mani che tremano—il dono della vita" (262) ["I bless the evening and the hour that they brought me, dying, to this house of your martyrdom and your faith to receive once again

---

38. Gabriele D'Annunzio, *La Gioconda*, in *Tragedie, sogni e misteri, Tutte le opere di Gabriele D'Annunzio*, ed. Egidio Bianchetti (Milan: Mondadori, 1964), 1:234.

from your hands—from these divine hands that tremble—the gift
of life"]. It is hoped that the life so transmitted will flow into
Lucio's hands, and Lorenzo Gaddi suggests a method by which the
transfer might be effected: "Quando Lucio riprenderà il suo lavoro,
dovrà il primo giorno modellare le vostre mani. Io ho un pezzo di
marmo antico, trovato negli Orti Oricellari. Glie lo darò, perché
le scolpisca in quello e poi le sospenda come un *ex-voto*" (239)
["When Lucio takes up his work again, he ought to model your
hands the first day. I have a piece of ancient marble, found in the
Oricellari Gardens. I will give it to him, that he might sculpt your
hands in it and hang it up as a votive offering"]. Such marble
hands, however, already exist in the text in the form of a copy of
a Verrocchio bust, indicated as one of the few props in the scene.
Silvia's hands are "of the same essence" as those of the bust:

> Sono perfette. Ricordate la donna del Verrocchio, la Donna
> dal mazzolino, quella dai capelli a grappoli? Ah, è là. . . .
> Voi avete dunque già riconosciuto la parentela. Quelle due
> mani sembrano consanguinee delle vostre, sono della mede-
> sima essenza. Vivono, è vero? d'una vita così luminosa che il
> resto della figura n'è oscurato. (*La Gioconda,* 239)

> [They are perfect. Remember the woman by Verrocchio, the
> woman with the bunch of flowers, the one with her hair in
> clusters? Ah, it is there. . . . Then you have already recog-
> nized the relationship. Those two hands seem of the same
> blood as yours, they are of the same essence. They are alive,
> aren't they, with a life so luminous that they overshadow the
> rest of the figure.]

The portrait bust is itself a synecdoche: it is not a representation
of a woman amputated from the waist down, but evokes the body
of which it is the partial representation. Here the hands have taken
on a life of their own, displacing the "whole" of which they are
"part." But that "whole" is itself a part, and the hands are a
synecdoche of synecdoche. The text seems to have entered into a
spiraling *mise en abîme* in which one synecdoche displaces another:
the gift of life passes from Silvia's hands to Lucio's hands to sculpted
hands to Silvia's hands. The catalogue could continue, one pair of

hands replacing another, one synecdoche handed over for another in a metaphorical relay.

The turns in the spiral trace the outlines of a reverse Pygmalion narrative. Silvia is on her way to becoming a statue, and her hands, already of the same essence as sculpted hands, will be the first to go. Though Lucio Settala himself will not mold her with *his* very own hands, he can be seen as an anti-Pygmalion. His desire is not to breathe life into his statues, not to give them a soul: "Io non scolpisco le anime" (274) ["I do not sculpt souls"], he says, expressing his aesthetic indifference to his wife's moral strength. This antiethical stance of the aesthete is hardly the sorrowful lament of a Pygmalion who longs for a soul for his creation, and it is Lucio's aesthetic ideal that will determine the kind of statue Silvia will become.

Lucio Settala's pseudo-Nietzschean aspiration to a realm beyond good and evil gives us no concrete idea of what that sculpted ideal might be, and there is, in fact, no direct description of his dazzling statue. Both the scene in which Silvia sees the statue for the first time and that in which she breaks the statue's fall take place behind a red curtain, offstage. It seems that she can be seen only obliquely, through allusive memory and feverish vision. Here the stage directions, never subordinate to dialogue in D'Annunzio's plays, are revealing. The entry to Lucio's studio is guarded by two Nikes, the Nike of Samothrace and the Paionios Nike, by fragments from the Panathenaic frieze, the bas-relief of Demeter from the Eleusis museum, the Ludovisian Medusa, and a small bronze Pegasus. It would seem that Lucio's ideal is Greek. But the "analogie di tutte le forme" ["analogies of all the forms"] go beyond those of antiquity and nationality: all except the Pegasus are fragments. The Nike of Samothrace is armless and headless; the Nike of Paionios handless, faceless, and wingless; the Panathenaic fragments are fragments of fragments; the bas-relief, a fragment; the Medusa, beheaded. The Pegasus, though presumably "whole," belongs to the series as a product of mutilation, born from the blood that sprang from the the Medusa's decapitation. The trait shared by all is mutilation. Lucio's aesthetic ideal is Greek, but "Greek" is here understood not as harmonius whole but as mutilated part.[39] If one considers

39. Though Maria Teresa Marabini-Moevs does not specifically address the

these fragments synecdoches, then according to Agamben's reasoning, they are already fetishistic and would negate the whole of which they were part as much as they evoke that whole.[40] Indeed, Greek art is known to us primarily as an art of fragments, of "mutilations" and "synecdoches" that are presumably parts of a once extant whole. We might say that it is difficult, if not impossible, to decide whether the aesthetic value of Greek sculpture—as mutilated fragment—can be accounted for by appealing to the imagined whole of which it is presumably a fragment, or whether their value does not lie instead in their mutilation. But the truly fetishistic quality of such fragments only emerges if we put in doubt the "whole" and ask: what if the Greeks only sculpted mutilated fragments to begin with? This seems to be the question posed by the text's refusal to represent the sculptor's "finished product." As we have noted, Lucio's own wondrously beautiful statue is never "seen"

grouping of these sculptures in *La Gioconda,* she suggests that the "analogy" that links them is not that of fragmentation but of adherent drapery, "that kind of drapery conventionally called *bagnato.*" Maria Teresa Marabini-Moevs, *Gabriele D'Annunzio e le estetiche della fine del secolo* (L'Aquila: L. V. Japadre, 1976), 222. This emphasis on drapery follows the standard art-historical description of these sculptures. That D'Annunzio was indeed appreciative of the clinging drapery is attested by the section of the *Taccuini* where he describes a statue of Victory by Paionios in the Acropolis Museum: "Il lungo peplo dorico disegna le forme nettamente come se fosse umido e aderisse alle membra vive. Tutto il marmo, se bene mutilato, è meraviglioso di audacia, di eleganza e di verità." *Taccuini, Tutte le opere di Gabriele D'Annunzio,* ed. Enrica Bianchetti (Verona: Mondadori, 1976), 53. ["The long Doric peplum traces the forms clearly as though it were damp and adhered to living members. Though mutilated, the marble statue is a marvel of audacity, elegance and truth."] Even here, however, mutilation appears as one of the statue's qualities, and it is above all the presence of a Medusa in *La Gioconda* that shifts the focus of the analogy. Read from the perspective of the 1898 tragedy, the 1895 annotations seem already to contain the (Greek) inspiration for *La Gioconda:* "la mano mutilata di Deidamia" ["the mutilated hand of Deidemia"] (53); "A destra del dio sta il re Enomaio, di cui non rimane se non il busto gagliardo e la testa mutilata" ["To the right of the god stands king Ennommus, of whom remains only a hearty bust and mutilated head"] (51); "Il braccio destro, che è monco, levava forse un grappolo. Dai ginocchi in giù mancano le gambe. . . . dei due piedi uno solo fu ritrovato" ["The right arm, which is handless, perhaps raised a bunch of grapes. The legs are missing from the knees down. . . . only one of two feet was found"] (50).

40. Though Agamben does suggest that fragments in general are fetishistic, he does not speak of Greek sculpture in particular.

in the text, but we do learn that it is a sphinx. According to the logic I have described, however, it is more "Greek" than Egyptian for its beauty lies in its mutilation: "imperiosa e pura che porta le ali imprigionate vive negli omeri" ["imperious and pure, with wings imprisoned alive in its shoulders"] it vividly recalls the "pesante mostro senza ali" ["heavy wingless monster"] that was its model. Lucio sculpts mutilations—a fact that does not bode well for Silvia, whose beautiful hands seem to be wings: "Sembra da qualche giorno che abbia le ali. . . . Sì, ella è veramente quali i vostri occhi di sorella la vedono. Esce dal suo martirio alata" (244) ["For several days now, it seems that she has wings. . . . Yes, she is truly as your sisterly eyes see her. She has emerged from martyrdom winged"]. Silvia emerged from martyrdom like a winged victory, but only mutilation can make her "Greek."[41] Both she and the statue are mutilated by its fall: she emerges handless, and her sister gathers up the severed hands to wrap them in the dampened cloth that had covered the clay statue; the statue emerges armless: "Così sul piedistallo sembra veramente un marmo antico, disseppellito in una delle Cicladi" (334) ["On the pedestal like that, it truly looks like an ancient marble, unearthed in one of the Cyclades"].

The fourth act reverses the reverse Pygmalion narrative of the first three acts: transformed into a "Greek" statue, the handless Silvia, "la mutilata," speaks. But this double reversal of the Pygmalion narrative is no longer Pygmalion at all, but instead its "consequence": the Medusan moment predicted by an earlier poem in the *Poema paradisiaco*.[42] The fourth act brings together a thematics of mutilation with what we might call a certain rhetorical destiny. Indeed, the inevitability of Silvia's fate, of her mutilation and petrification, is already inscribed in the poem, "Le mani" ["Hands"], an exercise in synecdoche in which the image of "la

41. Silvia's transformation into a wingless victory has been noted by Armand Caraccio: "Throughout the fourth act, Silvia Settala will carry her poor painful stumps like a wingless Victory, like a 'mutilated Victory'—whence the title of the trilogy." See Armand Caraccio, *D'Annunzio dramaturge* (Paris: Presses Universitaires de France, 1950), 75.

42. "In terms of mythological *exempla*," writes John Freccero, "petrification by the Medusa is the real consequence of Pygmalion's folly." See John Freccero, "Medusa: The Letter and the Spirit," *Dante: The Poetics of Conversion* (Cambridge: Harvard University Press, 1986), 130.

mutilata" first appears. A cataloguing of women's hands sets in
motion the mutilation intrinsic to catachrestic synecdoche and
culminates in a parenthetical, oneiric vision:

> (Nel sogno sta la mutilata, e attira.
>
> Nel sogno immobilmente eretta vive
> l'atroce donna da le mani mozze.
> E innanzi a lei rosseggiano due pozze
> di sangue, e le mani entro ancòra vive
> sonvi, neppure d'una stilla sozze.)[43]

[In dream stands the mutilated one, and attracts. In dream
immobily erect lives the atrocious woman with amputated
hands. And before her two pools of blood glow red, and the
hands therein are still alive, sullied by not even a drop of
blood.]

A parenthesis may qualify, explain, or be in apposition to the
syntactic construction it interrupts; here the "interruption" appears
to be an explanation and unfolding of the rhetorical figure upon
which the poem plays. What appears as an aside is in fact central
to the poem, for it is a literalization of that figure. If the part stands
for the whole in synecdoche, here the part(s) stand quite literally
before the (mutilated) whole. Like the hands of the Verrocchio
bust, they have taken on a life of their own ("ancòra vive"). All the
other hands in the poem are, by analogy, similarly severed. It is
not coincidental, then, that the lines immediately preceding the
parenthesis describe alabastrine hands as "più possenti di qualunque
spira":

> Altre (o le stesse?), mani alabastrine
> ma più possenti di qualunque spira,
> ci diedero un furor geloso, un'ira
> folle; e pensammo di mozzarle al fine.

43. Gabriele D'Annunzio, "Le mani," *Poema paradisiaco,* in *Versi d'amore e di gloria,* 1:684.

[Others (or the same?), alabastrine hands, but more powerful
than any coil, gave us a jealous furor, a mad ire; and we
thought of cutting them off at the end.]

These hands provoke a "furor geloso, un'ira folle" and a desire to
cut them off. The "spira," a coil of snakes, brings to mind the
Medusa's coiffure; the atrocious woman's attraction ("sta . . . e
attira), the Medusa's apotropaic power to fascinate and repel; her
stance ("immobilmente eretta"), the petrification of the observer.[44]
The parenthesis is thus the fulfillment of this desire and, by separat-
ing the "mutilata" from the rest of the poem, iconically mimes the
separation of part from whole. That is to say, the parenthesis
exhibits in its own structure the very structure it describes.

The final, supplementary act of *La Gioconda* occupies this same
parenthetical, oneiric space created in "Le mani." Considered thematically, the narrative can be said to move from cause to effect,
from Silvia's "sin" (another *fallo?*) to her punishment. From that
point of view the final act appears excessive, "tacked on," as it
were. From the point of view of fetishism, however, that narrative
can be said to move from effect to cause, from the fetishization of
hands to the "source" of the fetish. From this second point of view,
the final act logically (in the logic of fetishism) precedes the first
three acts, for it enacts a discovery of "mutilation." Like his reading
of Oedipus, D'Annunzio's reading of Medusa is a scrambling of
the Freudian code. For Freud of course, the terror of Medusa is "a
terror of castration that is linked to the sight of something."[45] The
final scene of *La Gioconda* is about nothing if not the "sight of
something" and that something is, as in Freud, perceived as an
absence. In both cases, that "sight of something" is the sight of
"nothing"; in this sense, neither is at odds with the false etymology
of the Medusa's name as "mé idòsan, quod videre non possit" ["that
which cannot be seen"].[46] For Freud that absence is the woman's
genitals or, more precisely, the "mother's penis"; the something
that is seen is seen as a negative and in that sense "cannot be seen."
For D'Annunzio, that absence is the "mother's hands," an absence

44. See Freud "Medusa's Head," 273–74.
45. Ibid., 273.
46. Noted in Freccero, 124.

that is hidden on stage and therefore cannot be seen. "La mutilata" is also "la castrata."

The scene plays upon the presence or absence of hands, upon the pathos of the twice-repeated disclosure of her mutilation, first to the childlike "La Sirenetta" and then to her daughter. While the first three acts focused on Silvia in her relation to Lucio, that is as wife, the final act focuses on Silvia in relation to Beata, that is as mother, as mother with something missing. A long-sleeved robe conceals her stumps, her clipped wings, but cannot conceal that there is something "lacking": "V'è nella sua movenza qualche cosa di manchevole, che suscita un'imagine vaga d'ali tarpate, che dà il sentimento vago d'una forza umiliata e tronca, d'una nobiltà avvilita, d'una armonia rotta." (*La Gioconda*, 316) ["There is something lacking in her movement; it calls up a vague image of clipped wings and creates a vague sense of a humiliated and trun-cated strength, of nobility brought low, of a broken harmony"]. Though Freud himself does not explicitly mention the Medusa in his essay on fetishism, her presence is implicit precisely as the horror of "qualche cosa di manchevole" which produces the fetishist's disavowal: "What happened, therefore, is that the boy refused to take cognizance of the fact of his having perceived that a woman does not have a penis. No, that could not be true. . . . the horror of castration has set up a memorial to itself in the creation of this substitute."[47] The fetish is thus a "memorial" dedicated to Medusa. The scenario of discovery and denial described by Freud is strikingly similar to the scene that takes place between Silvia and La Sirenetta:

Silvia Settala: Non le ho più.
La Sirenetta: Non le hai più! Te le hanno tagliate? Sei
    monca? No, no, no! Non è vero. Dimmi che non è
    vero.
Silvia Settala: Non le ho più.
La Sirenettta: Perché? perché?
Silvia Settala: Non dimandare!
(*La Gioconda*, 325)

[Silvia Settala: I don't have them anymore.

47. Freud, "Fetishism," 153–54.

La Sirenetta: You don't have them anymore? Have they cut
   them off? No hands? No, no, no! It isn't true. Tell me
   that it isn't true.
Silvia Settala: I don't have them anymore.
La Sirenetta: Why? Why?
Silvia Settala: Don't ask!]

La Sirenetta, of course, does not become a fetishist as a result of
her discovery, though she does reevoke the presence of her hands
in a nostalgic catalogue of their former functions ("me ne ricordo:
le vedo, le vedo" [325]) ["I remember them, I see them, I see
them"]. As in the case of *fallo*, what occurs here is not a matter of
a character who creates a fetish but rather of the text itself that
creates a fetish effect by setting up a tension between a multiplication of hands and their absence. The scene is filled with reminders
so blatant as to seem fingers pointing to her lack: the Verrocchio
bust, "le cui belle mani sono pur sempre intatte" ["whose beautiful
hands are still intact"], is once again present in the set description,
as is a spinet, "strumento abbandonato" ["abandoned instrument"].
La Sirenetta offers Silvia a five-fingered starfish, "più grande di una
mano" ["larger than a hand"], whose regenerative ability contrasts
almost sadistically with Silvia's condition. The presence of hands
pointing to the absence of hands is riveting (one could imagine
that, when the play is staged, the audience would fasten its attention upon the long sleeves, eager to catch a glimpse of the absence
of hands). The proliferation of such reminders can be compared
to Medusa's serpentine hair, for Freud suggests that it is the
"multiplication of penis symbols (that) signifies castration" and
mitigates the horror of discovery.[48] Already in Freud's recuperation
of these snakes as "mitigation," the logic of fetishism is at work,
suggesting that Medusa's head itself is a fetish.[49] The sight of
something that is a sight of nothing is already a fetishistic moment.

48. Freud, "Medusa's Head," 273.
49. Bernard Pautrat suggests that Medusa's head can be read as the extreme
example of a fetish in which castration is almost completely recognized: "Medusa's head is thus entirely paradoxical. At once an image of castration (open
mouth, eyes popping out of their sockets [regard exorbité]) and multiplied
image of the threatened penis. . . . It is a very paradoxical figuration, since the
Medusa carries on her face *at once castration and its denial*. . . . Medusa's head

The final act maintains a suspension between proliferation and absence by refusing to represent Beata's—the daughter's—recognition of her mother's mutilation. The scene, and hence the play, ends with the reunion of mother and daughter after months of separation caused by Silvia's convalescence. Beata brings flowers, which her mother cannot grasp, and expects caresses, which her mother cannot give.[50]

La voce di Beata: Mamma! Mamma! Mamma!
Silvia Settala: Beata! Beata!
Beata: Ah, quanto ho corso, quanto ho corso! Sono
    fuggita, sola. Ho corso, ho corso ... Non volevano
    lasciarmi venire. Ah, ma io sono fuggita, col mio fascio
    di fiori.
Silvia Settala: Sei tutta molle di sudore, sei tutta calda,
    bruci ... Mio Dio!
Beata: Perché non mi prendi? Perché non mi stringi?
    Prendimi! Prendimi, mamma!
Silvia Settala: Beata!
Beata: Non vuoi? Non vuoi?
Silvia Settala: Beata!
Beata: Tu giochi? Che nascondi? Oh, dammi, dammi
    quello che nascondi!
Silvia Settala: Beata! Beata!
Beata: Io t'ho portato i fiori, tanti fiori. Vedi? Vedi? Oh,
    la Sirenetta! Sei là? Vedi quanti? Tutti per te! Tieni!
Silvia Settala: Beata! Beata!
Beata: Non li vuoi? Prendi! Tieni!

faithfully obeys this logic of the fetish: simply, in it, reality outweighs desire; it is the recognition of castration that overwhelmingly dominates the denial; it is the absence of the penis being read before the fiction of its presence. If one were to read Medusa's head as a fetish, it would be the extreme example of a fetish in which castration is *almost* absolutely recognized and nevertheless immediately compensated for, obliterated by several substitutes: snakes, the head itself erected like a sun against the night of the abyss." See his "Nietzsche Médusé," *Nietzsche aujourd'hui?* (Paris: Union Générale d'Editions, 1973), 1:26–27.

    50. The offering of flowers, of course, recalls once again the Verrocchio bust *The Lady with a Bunch of Flowers.*

Silvia Settala: Beata!
Beata: Piangi? Piangi?
(*La Gioconda*, 336–39)

[Beata's voice: Mama! Mama! Mama!
Silvia Settala: Beata! Beata!
Beata: Oh, how I ran, how I ran! I ran off, all alone. I
    ran, I ran. They didn't want to let me come. Oh, but I
    ran away, with my bunch of flowers.
Silvia Settala: You are all damp with sweat, you are hot,
    burning ... Oh God!
Beata: Why don't you pick me up? Why don't you hug
    me? Pick me up, pick me up, Mama!
Silvia Settala: Beata!
Beata: Don't you want to? Don't you want to?
Silvia Settala: Beata!
Beata: Are you playing? What are you hiding? Oh, give
    me, give me what you are hiding!
Silvia Settala: Beata! Beata!
Beata: I brought you flowers, so many flowers! Do you see?
    See? Oh, Sirenetta! Are you there? See how many! All
    for you! Take them!
Silvia Settala: Beata! Beata!
Beata: Don't you want them? Take them! Take them!
Silvia Settala: Beata!
Beata: Are you crying? Are you crying?]

Silvia cannot give Beata what she hides, nor can the play end with
Silvia raising her arms so that her stumps are revealed. Such a
revelation would put an end to the fetishist's oscillation and lead
to a direct recognition of "castration."[51] In its place, we find a
displaced, and fetishistic revelation: this second disclosure is a

---

51. See Kofman, "Ça cloche," especially 132–39, and the text upon which
she comments, Derrida, *Glas*. See also Elizabeth Berg's review of Kofman,
"The Third Woman," *Diacritics* 12 (1982):11–20, and Naomi Schor, "Female
Fetishism: The Case of George Sand," in *The Female Body in Western Culture:
Contemporary Approaches*, ed. Susan Suleiman (Cambridge: Harvard University
Press, 1986), 363–72.

disclosure manqué. Thematically it describes the reunion of mother and child. Rhetorically, however, the final scene is a series of repetitions of single words and groups of words known as *geminatio*, a figure that, according to Heinrich Lausberg, is an emphatic expression of *separation* between people.[52] Mother and child are thus separated in their moment of reunion. It is not too farfetched to see in their separation a repetition of the earlier separation of part from whole. Such an interpretation is made possible not by a ideology that sees the child as part of the mother but by reading between the lines. It is literally between the lines, in the stage directions, that the amputation is reenacted: Silvia falls to her knees before her daughter and "un fiotto di pianto, che sgorga dagli occhi come il sangue da una ferita, le inonda la faccia" (339) ["a flood of tears, which burst from her eyes like blood from a wound, bathes her face"]. It is as though her wound were reopened, the hands severed again. But what we "see" is not the wound itself but the hands: in the final sentence of the play, hands once again appear on the ground before Silvia: "La Sirenetta, caduta anch'ella in ginocchio, prona, tocca con la fronte e con le palme distese la terra" (339) ["La Sirenetta, who has also fallen to her knees, prone, touches the earth with her forehead and with the palms of her hands spread wide"]. Just as Giuliana's "wound" was continually reopened, so must Silvia regain her hands in order to lose them again. The metaphorical relay in which one synecdoche is handed over for another is thus perpetuated, and must be perpetuated; the fetishistic synecdoche does not "refer" to a whole, to the thing itself, but only to other synecdoches. The text is caught in a loop and can only turn back upon itself: it must execute the same series

52. See Heinrich Lausberg, *Elemente der literarischen Rhetorik* (Munich: Max Hueber, 1963), par. 248: "*Geminatio* at the end [of a sentence] occurs as the insistent expression of spatial separation between people." Lanham's example of *geminatio* is equally appropriate: "O horror, horror, horror!" Lanham does not mention separation in his definition and cites only the repetition of the word *horror*, without including the context from which it is drawn. That context, however, is Macduff's reaction to the discovery of Duncan's murder in *Macbeth* (2.3.76–78), a sight compared to that of the Gorgon. See Richard Lanham, *A Handlist of Rhetorical Terms* (Berkeley: University of California Press, 1969), 46. It should be noted that Silvia says nothing other than "Beata." This repetition of her child's name, "blessed one," thus seems to take on a hortatory force as though the mother were blessing her child: "May you be blessed!"

of commands with no hope of exit, for only the Medusa's memorials can be seen, never the Medusa herself.

Indeed, once this mechanism has been revealed, we can reread the text and discover other memorials to Medusa. All, including Gioconda Dianti, are under the rule of synecdoche and participate in the Medusan moment that is this Pygmalion's lot. Like her namesake, La Gioconda's whole is in fact a "part"; just as the Mona Lisa's smile has taken on a life of its own, obscured the rest of the painting, so La Gioconda's gaze has taken over her "whole":

> La vita degli occhi è lo sguardo, questa cosa indicibile, più espressiva d'ogni parola, d'ogni suono, infinitamente profonda e pure istantanea come il baleno, più rapida ancora del baleno, innumerevole, onnipossente: insomma *lo sguardo*. Ora imagina diffusa su tutto il corpo di lei la vita dello sguardo. . . . Imagina questo mistero su tutto il suo corpo! Imagina per tutte le sue membra dalla fronte al tallone, questo apparire di vite fulminee! Potrai tu scolpire lo sguardo? Gli antichi accecarono le statue. Ora—imagina—tutto il corpo di lei è come lo sguardo. . . . Te l'ho detto: mille statue, non una. La sua bellezza vive in tutti i marmi. (274–75)

> [The life of the eyes is the gaze, this unspeakable thing, more expressive than any word, than any sound, infinitely profound and yet instantaneous as a flash, even swifter than a flash, innumerable, omnipotent: in a word, the *gaze*. Now imagine the life of the gaze diffused all over her body. . . . Imagine this mystery over all her body! Imagine over all her limbs from her forehead to her heel this lightning flash of lives! Could you sculpt that gaze? The ancients blinded their statues. Now, imagine, her entire body is like the gaze. . . . I have told you: a thousand statues, not one. Her beauty lives in all marbles.]

La Gioconda's beauty is dazzling; the multiplication of the gaze ("questa cosa . . . innumerevole") not only recalls the multiplication of hands in the final act and the multiplication of serpents on Medusa's head but evokes a "blinding" at its center: "Gli antichi accecarono le statue." La Gioconda is already a blinding and blinded statue.[53] Indeed, La Gioconda's attraction is a stony one; when Lucio sees her, he sees marble: "Quando mi apparve l'altra, io pensai a tutti i blocchi di marmo contenuti nelle cave delle montagne lontane" (274) ["When the other woman appeared to me, I thought of all the blocks of marble contained in the caves of the

53. This description of La Gioconda parallels, not coincidentally, Rilke's description of the "Archaïscher Torso Apollos" in the *Neue Gedichte*. That Rilke knew the play is made evident by his writings on Rodin, where he alludes to Eleonora Duse's portrayal of Silvia in *La Gioconda*. This mention appears precisely in the context of a discussion of sculpture (Rodin's *La méditation*) and of "mutilation" as aesthetic ideal: "The arms are noticeably absent. Rodin felt them in this instance to be something extraneous to the body, which sought to be its own concealment, without external aid. One recalls Duse, how in one of D'Annunzio's plays, when left bitterly alone, she attempts to give an armless embrace, to hold without hands. This scene, in which her body learns a caress far beyond its natural scope, belongs to the unforgettable moments of her acting. It conveyed the impression that arms were a superfluous adornment, something for the rich and self-indulgent, something which those in the pursuit of poverty could easily cast aside. She looked in that moment not like a person lacking something important; but rather like someone who has given away his cup that he may drink from the stream itself, like someone who is naked and a little helpless in his absolute nakedness. The same effect is produced by the armless statues of Rodin; nothing essential is lacking. We stand before them as before something whole and complete, which allows of no addition. The feeling of incompleteness does not come from the mere aspect of a thing, but is due to elaborate reflexion, to petty pedantry, which says that where there is a body there must be arms, that a body without arms can, in no instance, be complete." The "petty pedantry" Rilke so eloquently describes is precisely the logic of Freud's infantile theorists of sexuality: where there is a body there must be a penis, and a body without a penis can, in no instance, be complete. Rilke's comparison of the Duse to Rodin's armless statues not only supports the argument that Silvia is turned into a statue, but puts into question the (synecdochal) relation of part to whole. Thus the "mutilated whole" becomes the harmonious, complete whole, while the severed "part" itself becomes another whole: "The artist has the right to make one thing out of many and a world out of the smallest part of a thing. Rodin has made hands, independent, small hands which, without forming part of a body are yet alive. Hands rising upright, angry and irritated, hands whose five bristling fingers seem to bark like the five throats of a Cerberus. Hands in motion, sleeping hands and hands in the act of awaking; criminal hands, weighted by heredity, hands that are tired and have lost all desire, lying like some sick beast crouched in a corner, knowing none can help them. . . . Hands have a history of their own, they have, indeed, their own civilization, their special beauty; we concede to them the right to have their own development, their own wishes, feelings, moods and favourite occupations." Rainer Maria

distant mountains"]. Her dazzling effect is similar to that of Lucio's feverish vision of his own creation:

> Nella prima febbre quando avevo ancòra il piombo nella carne e il rombo continuo della morte su l'anima perdita, la vedevo dritta a pié del letto, accesa come una torcia, come se io medesimo l'avessi plasmata in una materia incandescendente. (252)

> [In the first fever when I still had the lead in my flesh and the continous rumble of death on my lost soul, I saw her erect at the foot of my bed, lit like a torch, as though I myself had molded her in incandescent matter.]

In his convalescence, he has lost the vision of his fiery statue and suggests that his reaction to seeing it again would be horror: "Non la vedo più. Mi sfugge. Appare e dispare come in un baleno, confusa. Se l'avessi ora qui davanti, mi parrebbe nuova; gitterei un grido" (251–52) ["I see her no longer. She escapes me. She appears and disappears as though in a flash, confused. If I had her here before me now, she would seem new; I would scream"]. The analogy between La Gioconda and Lucio's statue, with its juxtaposition of La Gioconda as all eyes and the statue as that which is unseen, offstage, *ab-scena*, and hence (etymologically) obscene, seems to be yet another memorial to Medusa. Lucio is surrounded by Medusas; no wonder then that, in the last mention of him in the play, he seems to have worked himself into a frenzy:

> Il suo viso è così scarno che sembra debba divorarglielo il fuoco dagli occhi. Quando parla, si eccita stranamente. Ne rimasi turbato. Lavora, lavora, lavora, con una terribile furia: forse cerca di sottrarsi a un pensiero che lo rode. (333)

> [His face is so emaciated that it seems the the fire of his eyes

Rilke, *Rodin and Other Prose Pieces*, trans. G. Craig Houston (New York: Quartet Books, 1986), 18–19. For an account of Rilke's relationship to D'Annunzio, see George Schoolfield, "Rilke and D'Annunzio: A Painful Case," *Quaderni Dannunziani* 3–4 (1988): 305–21.

must be devouring it. When he speaks, he becomes strangely agitated. It troubled me. He works, he works, he works, with a terrible fury. Perhaps he is trying to evade a thought that gnaws at him.}

The terrible "fury" with which he works is a fury's sister, the Gorgon ("lavora, lavora, lavora"—yet another *geminatio* that recalls Lanham's example: "O horror, horror, horror"). We can only speculate about the thought that eats away at him.

The thought that eats away at the text, however, is clear: the Medusan moment is the consequence of the decadent's occupation of the woman's body, of his appropriation of physical alterity as a figure for psychic alterity. Just as discussions of the androgyny of genius and poetic production were haunted by figures of physiological monstrosity, so is the desire for eviration haunted by its physiological "realization." In order for that desire to perpetuate itself, such a realization must remain suspended by the fetishist's disavowal. If *La Gioconda* is taken as the outcome and culmination of the decadent texts discussed here, then we can say that the "degenderation" they propose is precariously suspended from the logic of castration: if "woman" is and is not castrated, then "man," too, is and is not castrated.[54] The "law" thereby transgressed is the law and logic of castration, and eroticism resonates from the fetishist's oscillation.

54. On fetishism as a "third way" out of the binary logic of castration, see Berg, 11–20.

Afterword   Alibis

In the fall of 1987, an episode of the television series *Cagney and Lacey* brought the problem of reading and writing about D'Annunzio to prime time. In this episode, the show's "good cops" go undercover in order to expose a crooked game-show host. Dressed as fruits and vegetables, they appear as contestants on the rigged quiz, where they are asked a number of "general knowledge" questions, among them "Who was Italy's first Fascist?" Confident, one of the cops promptly answers: "Benito Mussolini." The buzzer sounds: wrong. Another try: "Gabriele D'Annunzio." Right. If this is "general knowledge" (and has filtered down to American popular culture), it is also perhaps the commonplace that has contributed most to blackening the screen that obscures our reading of D'Annunzio, and it may thus a priori color readings of this book as well. I would like, then, in conclusion, briefly to address this question with an eye to future work.

No rhetorical strategy is in itself either politically progressive or reactionary. In the hands of Baudelaire, Nietzsche, and D'Annunzio, the nineteenth-century rhetoric of sickness opens onto the discovery of the unconscious and the exploration of psychic alterity which underlie the "decentering of the subject"; in the hands of Lombroso, it opens onto twentieth-century theories of racial purity. Degenerates and "degenderates" are equally condemned by fascism and nazism, and "health" reappears as a national, and in the case of nazism, racial ideal. From this point of view, the literary texts I have analyzed can be held to be in the proto-Fascist camp only if all aspects of modernism itself are held to be proto-Fascist. But at such a level of generality, protofascism no longer has any specificity at all, either ideologically or historically; it becomes merely a term that refers to that which chronologically preceded fascism.

This problem is compounded by the fact that "Fascist ideology" and "Fascist philosophy" have been viewed as oxymorons, as contradictions in terms.[1] This denial of the existence of a Fascist ideology has roots in the political condemnation of fascism; to recognize an ideology or philosophy in fascism would be to dignify it with an intellectual and theoretical stature it does not merit. And by bringing with it the problem of consent, such recognition would also threaten the notion that fascism was nothing other than state violence imposed upon a fundamentally anti-Fascist people.[2] The political usefulness (and, at a certain historical moment, perhaps even necessity) of this move is clear: if fascism has no ideology, then it becomes easier to close that particular "parenthesis in history" (as Croce called it), and to consider fascism a historical aberration. Historians have thus often resorted to chronological definitions of fascism itself. Edward Tannenbaum's solution is typical: "The word Fascism with a capital 'F' refers specifically to the political system of Italy from the early 1920s through the early 1940s and should not be a problem; the problem concerns the word fascism with a small 'f.'"[3] The "problem" is thus displaced onto "fascism." But if we are to know what is "proto-Fascist" in Italy, we must also know what is Fascist with a capital "F," and defining *both* chronologically empties them of any sense they might have in reference to the ideology of a text: how, indeed, can one look for the ideological roots of something that presumably has no ideology? I should emphasize here that I am speaking of *Italian* fascism (and of studies of Italian fascism), not of French fascism, where fascism-as-movement never solidified into fascism-as-regime, or of nazism, in which anti-Semitism was a constitutive element.[4]

1.   For an excellent discussion of this view, see Pier Giorgio Zunino, *L'ideologia del fascismo: Miti, credenze e valori nella stabilizzazione del regime* (Bologna: Il Mulino, 1985), especially 11–62.

2.   Ibid., 14–24.

3.   Edward Tannenbaum, *The Fascist Experience: Italian Society and Culture* (New York: Basic Books, 1972), 3.

4.   Because French fascism never became a regime, it has seemed a particularly "pure" case. Zeev Sternhell writes that "ideologies and movements may be

Distinctions need to be made, and *are* made by scholars such as Renzo De Felice, Zeev Sternhell, or George Mosse.[5] It is not, for example, of small importance that anti-Semitism and racism were not an integral part of Italian fascism, which, as De Felice writes, "adopted them late and largely for reasons of political convenience and to avoid being at odds with other Axis powers."[6] As a result of those distinctions, however, studies of French Fascist ideology or of Nazi ideology cannot automatically be transferred to Italian fascism, and it is only relatively recently, above all with the work of Renzo De Felice, that studies of Italian fascism have begun to allow us to understand the specificity of *its* ideology. That work of description and analysis of Fascist ideology must be continued not only by historians but also by literary scholars before we can "judge" the culture that produced fascism and the culture that fascism produced.

Indeed, in the absence of an analysis of Fascist ideology, the attribution of protofascism to D'Annunzio has had more to do with retrospective reading than with whatever antidemocratic, antiparliamentary statements we might (and can) isolate in his works. This reading is based on the biographical D'Annunzio, who in 1919 occupied Fiume and as the *comandante* acquired a political following and stature that for a brief period rivaled Mussolini's. Mussolini himself adopted slogans and certain elements of his political style from D'Annunzio and took it upon himself to ensure D'Annunzio's continued assent, or at least silence, during the regime.[7] It is from this final period of his

discovered in their purest form" before coming to power and that France therefore "offers especially suitable conditions" for the study of Fascist ideology. See Sternhell, *Neither Right nor Left: Fascist Ideology in France*, trans. David Maisel (Berkeley: University of California Press, 1986), 1; see also Alice Y. Kaplan, *Reproductions of Banality: Fascism, Literature, and French Intellectual Life* (Minneapolis: University of Minnesota Press, 1986), 51–55.

5. This is not to say that common denominators cannot be found. For concise discussions of the need for such distinction, see Renzo De Felice, *Intervista sul fascismo*, ed. Michael Ledeen (Bari: Laterza, 1976), and De Felice, *Interpretations of Fascism*, trans. Barbara Huff Everett (Cambridge: Harvard University Press, 1977), especially the chapter "Fascism as a Problem of Interpretation."

6. De Felice, *Interpretations of Fascism*, 11.

7. On D'Annunzio in Fiume, see Renzo De Felice, *D'Annunzio politico* (Bari: Laterza, 1978); De Felice, *Sindacalismo rivoluzionario e fiumanesimo nel carteggio*

life that D'Annunzio earned the epithet "the John the Baptist" of fascism or, as Michael Ledeen puts it, "the first Duce." From that point, his works will be reread on the assumption that biographical continuity is equal to, indeed causes, an ideological continuity and coherence in an author's texts. But drawing literary conclusions from biographical data, like drawing biographical conclusions from literary data, depends on elision and an ignorance of the rhetorical nature of the literary text. Either tactic may be useful for indicting or absolving authors and their works, but neither helps us to understand the texts in question. I do not mean to indict or to absolve. A reading of D'Annunzio's writings and speeches during the Fiume period does indeed have much to tell us about fascism-as-movement; revolutionary elements still coexist with the reactionary elements that reigned when fascism becames regime. Such a reading will also tell us what Mussolini and fascism could absorb from D'Annunzio and what turned out to be indigestible.[8] Fascism incorporates

---

De Ambris—D'Annunzio (1919–1922) (Brescia: Morcelliana, 1966); De Felice, *Mussolini il rivoluzionario, 1883–1920* (Turin: Einaudi, 1965); and Michael Ledeen, *The First Duce: D'Annunzio at Fiume* (Baltimore: Johns Hopkins University Press, 1977).

8. The Fascists themselves were careful to establish a proper distance from D'Annunzio at the same time as they attempted to win over his followers. In the entry "Fascism" in the 1932 *Enciclopedia Treccani* (the first section of which is signed "Benito Mussolini" but was presumably written by Giovanni Gentile, and the second half of which is signed "Gioacchino Volpe"), a line is carefully drawn between D'Annunzio and Fiume, and Mussolini and fascism. Volpe writes of the November 1921 Congress of Fascists: "For four or five months, there had been a word that agitated souls and created oppositions between the men most representative of fascism, almost between city and city, region and region: the peace treaty. There were the relationships between Fascists and the Legionnaires of Fiume, between fascism and D'Annunzianism, a little bit between Mussolini and D'Annunzio, who watched over his young companions from afar. Not all of 'Fiumeanism' [*fiumanesimo*] had mixed into fascism. A part of it [Fiumeanism] had become a supporter of the word of Carnaro, almost opposed to the word of fascism. . . . [Mussolini] had words of gratitude for D'Annunzio's work, but excluded the possibility that fascism would find its laws in the statutes of Carnaro: he admitted only that these latter had been animated by a spirit that the Fascists could absorb and make their own." The "word of Carnaro" here refers to the constitution that D'Annunzio and Alceste De Ambris had written for Fiume, the "Carta del Carnaro." Among the words of Carnaro which Mussolini did not make his own was women's suffrage. *Enciclopedia italiana*, ed. Istituto

ideologically incompatible elements from diverse literary and philosophical sources and musters considerable rhetorical force to produce a semblance of coherence, but not everything can be incorporated and certainly not D'Annunzio's entire corpus.

I have here attempted to go behind the blackened screen of retrospective reading and to analyze the decadent rhetoric of sickness in the late nineteenth century. This rhetoric of sickness provided the occasion and alibi for an alterity that positivism labeled criminal, that literary critics have found offensive, and that fascism, with its celebration of virility, found indigestible. While this rhetoric may be no alibi for D'Annunzio's later political involvement, it points to a D'Annunzio whose texts are embedded in quite a different context, quite another matrix. If the decadents' "occupation" is dependent on the expulsion of woman from the scene of art, it also refuses the logic of castration which would assign her the place of "have-not" in a world of haves and have-nots. Attended by furies, chimeras, androgynes, hermaphrodites, and Medusas, that project is tormented and fraught with contradictions and is part of what Christine Buci-Glucksmann has called "the feminization of culture" in the second half of the nineteenth century and the beginning of the twentieth, "a great labor of deconstruction of the frontier of masculine and feminine identities," a labor in which "the metaphor of the feminine arises as an element of rupture of a certain rationality put into question, of a historical and symbolic continuum, by designating a heterogeneity and a new alterity."[9] The rationality it calls into question is that of positivism and all ideologies of "progress"; the symbolic continuum, that of the figuration of sexual difference. In appropriating

G. Treccani (Milan: Rizzoli, 1932), 14:859. For a discussion of the Fiumean writings, see Barbara Spackman, "'Il verbo (e)sangue': Gabriele D'Annunzio and the Ritualization of Violence," *Quaderni d'Italianistica* 4.2 (1983): 219–29; and Spackman, "The Fascist Rhetoric of Virility," *Stanford Italian Review* 8.1–2 (1988): 81–101.

9. Christine Buci-Glucksmann, *La raison baroque: De Baudelaire à Benjamin* (Paris: Galilée, 1984), 33. I learned of this fine book (whose reading of Baudelaire is complementary to my own) only after completing my manuscript, and am grateful to Linda Bolis for bringing it to my attention. For an extended critique of the appropriation of the position of woman by contemporary "male" theory, see Alice Jardine, *Gynesis: Configurations of Woman and Modernity* (Ithaca: Cornell University Press, 1985).

and speaking of, through, and for the otherness of woman's body, these writers place themselves "elsewhere" on the continuum of sexual difference, and sickness provides them with the alibi they need for an alterity that positivism finds criminal. But the expulsion and exclusion of woman from this scene is also the mark of a nonrecognition of the "other"; it is this expulsion that comes back to haunt the text in the form of La Gioconda's stony gaze. The fetishist's disavowal thus can be taken as an alibi in yet another sense: it is the excuse for that nonrecognition, a claim to have been elsewhere than at the scene in which diversity is transformed into difference. It is a precarious position, which, on the one hand, can fall into appropriation and yet, on the other, refuses the opposition that makes such appropriation possible. I hope to have shown not only how these texts fall into appropriation but also how, in their most precarious moments, they potentially resist insertion into the symbolic continuum that has defined woman as man's other.

Index

Library of Congress Cataloging-in-Publication Data

Spackman, Barbara, 1952–
    Decadent genealogies: the rhetoric of sickness from Baudelaire to D'Annunzio /
Barbara Spackman.
        p.   cm.
    Includes index.
    ISBN 0-8014-2290-6 (alk. paper)
    1. Decadence (Literary movement) 2. Decadence in literature. 3. Mental illness in
literature. 4. Literature, Modern—19th century—History and criticism.
5. Literature, Modern—20th century—History and criticism. 6. Literature—
Psychological aspects. I. Title.
PN56.D45S63   1989   809'.93353—dc20   89-7303

3995 9I DUP
3995

895